PRACTICE OF PSYCHOSEXUAL MEDICINE

Selected papers from the First International
Conference on Psychosexual Medicine

7–10 July 1982
Brighton

and other meetings of the
Institute of Psychosexual Medicine

PRACTICE OF PSYCHOSEXUAL MEDICINE

Editor
KATHARINE DRAPER
Institute of Psychosexual Medicine

John Libbey: London

ACKNOWLEDGEMENTS

My thanks are due to the authors, who gave permission for their papers to be used in this book; to Dr I. C. Barne and Dr Fay Hutchinson who, as Programme Secretaries of the IPM, arranged the meetings at which they were given; to Miss Valerie Thompson, FRCOG, who edited the transcripts of these meetings and prepared a bibliography; to the Postgraduate Education Department of Wyeth Pharmaceuticals Ltd, who funded the printing of the transcripts of the weekend meetings; to Dr Robina Thexton for assistance in selecting the Seminar Transcript; to Mrs Mary Walford for her indefatigable typing; to Mrs Mary Edwards for her skilled editorial assistance; to the *British Journal of Sexual Medicine* for permission to republish the following papers: Postpartum Sexuality, K. Draper (pp. 112–115); Pre-hysterectomy States, T. F. Main (pp. 122–125); Impotence: Fifty Cases, J. Berry and J. Yorston (pp. 136–144); and Retarded Ejaculation, R. Lincoln and R. Thexton (pp. 151–155); to Dr R. Sampson, who edited the papers from the Brighton Conference; to Miss P. Draper, who compiled the Index; and last, but not least, to my family for tolerating my distraction during the compilation of the book.

British Library Cataloguing in Publication Data:

Practice of Psychosexual medicine: selected papers
  from the first International Conference on
  Psychosexual Medicine, 7–10 July, 1982, Brighton and
  other meetings of the Institute of Psychosexual
  Medicine
  1. Sex (Psychology)—Congresses
  I. Draper, Katharine   II. International
  Conference on Psychosexual Medicine (*1st: 1982: Brighton*)
  155.3'4   BF692

  ISBN 0-86196-020-3

First published 1983 by

John Libbey & Company Limited
80–84 Bondway, London SW8 1SF

Printed in Great Britain by
Whitstable Litho Ltd., Whitstable, Kent

Contributors

(*Member of the Institute of Psychosexual Medicine)

*DOREEN M. M. ANDERSON MB, ChB: SCMO Family Planning and Psychosexual Clinics, Wakefield; 4 Newstead Road, St Johns, Wakefield, Yorkshire.

AGNES BEGG: SCMO Family Planning Services, Edinburgh; 7 Malta Terrace, Edinburgh, EH4 1HR.

*JANE BERRY MB, ChB, DA (deceased): SCMO Community Health, Family Planning and Psychosexual Problems, Winchester, Hampshire.

*JUNE BETTS MB, BS, MRCOG: Clinical Assistant, Charing Cross Hospital, London, W6; 59c North Street, Carshalton, Surrey.

JULES BLACK MB, BS, MRCOG, FRACOG: Obstetrician/Gynaecologist/Sexologist; 253 Oxford Street, Bondi Junction, Sydney, New South Wales, Australia.

*MARGARET BLAIR MB, BS (deceased): Associate Specialist, Charing Cross Hospital, London, W6.

*JAMES BRADSHAW MA, MRCOG: Consultant Gynaecologist/Obstetrician, Duchess of Kent Military Hospital, Catterick Garrison, N. Yorks; 18 Abbey Road, Darlington, Co. Durham.

*H. MORAG BRAMLEY MA, MB, ChB: SCMO, Genitourinary and Psychosexual Clinics, The Royal Hallamshire Hospital, Sheffield; Green Hills, Back Lane, Hathersage, Sheffield, S30 1AR.

K. B. CHINOY MD, FRCS, MRCOG: Obstetrician/Gynaecologist; 921 Garfield, Suite 3, Topeka, Kansas 66606, USA.

*ELPHIS CHRISTOPHER MB, BS, DObst, RCOG, DCH: SCMO Family Planning, Haringey Health Authority, Tottenham Town Hall, The Green, London, N15.

*RUTH E. COLES MB, ChB: Medical Director, Avon Brook Advisory Service; 21 Richmond Hill, Clifton, Bristol.

*JOAN R. COOMBS MB, ChB: SCMO Psychosexual Clinics in Leeds and Bradford; 13 Holly Park, Huby, Leeds, Yorkshire.

*ELAINE COOPER MB, ChB, MRCS, LRCP: Central Health Clinic and Domiciliary Family Planning, Southampton; 15 Richmond Gardens, Portswood, Southampton, SO2 1RY.

*S. A. CORRIN MB, BS, LRCP, MRCS, DObst, RCOG: SCMO Lewisham and North Southwark Health Authority; 14 Foxgrove Road, Beckenham, Kent.

*ELIZABETH J. DEMAN MRCS, LRCP, DObst, RCOG: Clinical Assistant, Fertility Clinic, Royal Free Hospital, Pond Street, London NW3.

*BARBARA DEVEREUX MB, BS: SCMO Family Planning and Psychosexual Clinics, Lowestoft and Norwich; 6 Glebe Close, Lowestoft, Suffolk, NR32 4NU.

*KATHARINE DRAPER MA, MB, BChir: SCMO Lewisham and North Southwark Health Authority; 29 High Street, Chipstead, Sevenoaks, Kent, TN13 2RW.

*ROLAND FREEDMAN MB, BChir, FRCGP: Practitioner/Lecturer in Family Medicine, University of Newcastle-upon-Tyne; 1 The Grove, Newcastle-upon-Tyne, NE3 1NU.

*MARGARET GILL MB, BS, MRCS, LRCP: Psychosexual Clinics, Lisson Grove Health Centre and East Hertfordshire; 10 Peters Wood Hill, Ware, Herts, SG12 9NR.

*JUDY GILLEY MB, BS: General Practitioner, Cornwall House, Cornwall Avenue, London N3.

*GILLIAN HINSHELWOOD MB, BS: Psychotherapy and Psychosexual Counsellor, Youth Advisory Centre, 26 Prince of Wales Road, London NW5; 24 Bramshall Gardens, London, NW5.

*FAY HUTCHINSON MB, BS, LMCC: Medical Officer in Charge, Brook Advisory Centre, 233 Tottenham Court Road, London, W1.

*FRANK SEYMOUR JOHNSON FRCOG, Dip Psychother, MB, BS: Consultant Gynaecologist/Obstetrician, Ashington Hospital, Northumberland; Fordwich House, Hepscott, Morpeth, Northumberland.

*JANE KILVINGTON MB, BS: Psychosexual Problems Clinics, Hertfordshire; 122 Marshalwick Lane, St Albans, Herfordshire.

*ELSIE KOADLOW: Consultant and Director of Sexual Counselling Clinic, Albert Street Medical Centre, 376 Albert Street, East Melbourne 3002, Australia.

*ROSEMARIE LINCOLN MB, BS: SCMO Norwich Health Authority and Norfolk and Norwich Hospital, 67 Yarmouth Road, Norwich, NR7 UWW.

D. C. MACDONALD BURNS MB, BS, LRCP, MRCOG: Consultant Venereologist, Royal Free Hospital, Pond Street, London, NW3.

*TOM MAIN MD, FRC Psych, FRANZCP, DPM: formerly Medical Director of The Cassel Hospital, Psychoanalyst in Private Practice; 6 Sherwood Close, Barnes, London, SW13 0JD.

*PETER MITFORD MB, BS, MRCGP: General Prctitioner; 6 Howard Road, Morpeth, Northumberland, NE61 1JE.

*DOROTHY MORGAN LRCP, MRCS: Principal Medical Officer, Powys Health Authority; Bellfountain Cottage, Crickhowell, Powys.

H. MUSAPH: Professor of Medical Sexology, Academisch Ziekenhuis Utrecht; Postbus 16250, 3500 CG Utrecht, Holland.

*JEAN PASMORE MRCS, LRCP: The Cassel Hospital (retired); South Cottage, Ham Gate Avenue, Ham Common, Richmond, Surrey.

S. E. PROCTOR MB, BS, MRC Psych: Senior Registrar in Psychiatry, Royal Victoria Infirmary, Newcastle-upon-Tyne; Hill House, Melbury Road, High Heaton, Newcastle-upon-Tyne, NE7 7DE.

*MARY REES MB, BS, DObst RCOG: Hon. Senior Registrar, Family Planning, Psychosexual and Infertility Clinics, Kings College Hospital, London SE5; 103 St Helens Park Road, Hastings, Sussex.

*PATRICIA ROBERTS MB, ChB: Visiting Psychotherapist, HM Prison, Maidstone, Kent; Rory Cottage, Taylors Lane, Trottiscliffe, Maidstone, Kent, ME19 5DS.

*RUTH SKRINE MB, ChB, MRCGP: Psychosexual Clinic, Bath; Castanea House, Sham Castle Lane, Bath, Somerset, BA2 6JN.

*ANNE V. SMITH MB, BS: General Practitioner; Shieldfield Health Clinic, Newcastle-upon-Tyne 2.

*ROBINA THEXTON MB, BS, LRCP, MRCS: Psychosexual Clinics for several London Health Authorities; 41 Hillcroft Crescent, Ealing, London, W5 2SG.

*ALEXANDRA TOBERT MB, BS, DCH: Lecturer in Psychosexual Medicine, The City Hospital, Nottingham; 2 Regent Street, Nottingham.

*PRUDENCE TUNNADINE MB, BS, DObst, RCOG: Private Practice and Director of Training, Institute of Psychosexual Medicine; 11 Chandos Street, Cavendish Square, London W1M 9DE.

*ELSPETH WILLIAMSON MB, BS, DCH: Genetic Counsellor; Department of Child Health, The General Hospital, Southampton.

*JESSIE YORSTON MD: SCMO Family Planning and Psychosexual Clinics, Winchester and Southampton; Luibeg, Gardiners Lane, Embley, Romsey, Hampshire.

DEDICATION

This book is dedicated to the memory of Margaret Blair, the first Secretary of the Institute of Psychosexual Medicine, and Chairman of the Council at the time of her death in June, 1982.

CONTENTS

OTHER SETTINGS

Introduction

Katharine Draper

Psychosexual medicine is the understanding of sexual anxiety wherever it presents. Doctors working in many different fields such as general practice, gynaecology, family planning, psychiatry, and genito-urinary medicine, are often confronted with patients who offer a psychosexual complaint which they feel ill-equipped to treat. This book describes the work of the Institute of Psychosexual Medicine (IPM) whose prime aim is to train doctors to respond to and work with patients with psychosexual anxieties in whatever guise they present.

The papers collected in this book have all been given since the IPM, founded in 1974, began to hold clinical meetings, but the origins of this work go back 25 years. It was in the clinics of the Family Planning Association (FPA), with their implicit acceptance of sexuality, that women first voiced their worries about sexual problems. In 1958, a number of doctors working in the FPA, sensitive to the women's distress but uncertain how to respond, asked the psychoanalyst Dr Michael Balint to provide training (Balint & Balint 1961). This request led him to form the first seminar of ten doctors who treated only cases of women with sexual difficulties in their family planning work. Balint's method of training combined study and research; only three years later a study of non-consummation was published: *Virgin Wives* (Friedman 1962). This was followed by findings on frigidity (Blair & Pasmore 1964).

Within two years more doctors had started seminar training with other psychoanalysts and eventually special marital problem clinics were set up at which couples presented; these findings were published in *Sexual Discord in Marriage* (Courtney 1962). Dr Main, now our President, led a seminar whose findings are described in *Contraception and Sexual Life* (Tunnadine 1970). As the demand for training grew some members of the original seminars were trained to lead other groups, and this method of training became defined and more widely available. When the clinical functions of the FPA were absorbed into the National Health Service in 1974, a group of doctors working in psychosexual medicine, supported by Mrs Nancy Raphael, decided to form the IPM which is now responsible for training and accreditation.

A doctor who undertakes training joins a basic seminar. When a group of doctors want to meet together for this purpose the Institute will provide a trained leader in most areas of the United Kingdom, and the seminars may be recognised under Section 63 for General Practitioners.

Doctors who seek to specialise in psychosexual medicine may continue their

1

training in an advanced seminar. After this they may offer themselves for examination by the Assessment Panel, and if successful they are awarded the Institute's Certificate of Competence in Psychosexual Medicine. A doctor so qualified is competent to accept referrals from other practitioners and agencies. Over 1300 doctors have now experienced basic training and over 400 have persisted in advanced seminars and presented themselves before the panel to become accredited as specialists in psychosexual medicine. Details of these regulations and of membership of the IPM are given in Appendix II.

In addition to the prime task of training, the IPM also holds clinical meetings, evening meetings in London and an annual weekend meeting at different locations in the provinces. These meetings are only open to members of the Institute but this year the first International Conference, open to all medical practitioners, was held at Brighton. When considering the publication of the proceedings of this conference it was decided to include papers which had been given at earlier meetings, but were only available to members of the Institute. Rather than arrange these papers chronologically under the meetings at which they had been presented, it was decided to regroup them according to topics, so that they make a statement of the work of the Institute.

The keystone of this book is the exposition of our method of training to increase skill rather than knowledge; this is followed by a transcript of a seminar and papers by a number of doctors on their own experiences of training and the way that this has affected their work. After this I have grouped together papers in which the method of working is discussed — including the differentiation from other forms of psychotherapy, the merits of treating couples, and the doctors' anxieties.

Although we seek, in each clinical encounter, to help the patients to discover for themselves the nature of the unique block that prevents them from enjoying and treating their individual instincts, we find that certain patterns of difficulty emerge. The insights that have been gained from working with patients are given in a collection of clinical papers. After some contributions on difficulties in presentation and consummation there are major papers and case studies on men's and women's problems. The details of the case studies have been amended to protect confidentiality.

Doctors who have developed an awareness of patients' sexual anxiety find that this also affects their work in other settings, giving them an increased insight into underlying conflicts which can aid their resolution. This is illustrated in a selection of papers from many different work situations including family planning, general practice, gynaecology and more unusual settings such as genetic counselling and work in prisons.

The papers that were given by members at the Brighton Conference have been included in the appropriate sections. The programme of the meeting, with the talks that set the scene and summarised the proceedings, are included, with the free communications, as Appendix I.

All the papers in this book were written for delivery at clinical meetings, not for publication in scientific journals, and this presentation has been largely retained. As well as the major papers, many short cases described by numerous different authors have been included. These papers illustrate the fact that the IPM is not

2

concerned only with training those who specialise in this field, but also with helping many doctors to work with increased understanding in their individual settings.

By the time the work of Masters & Johnson (1970) and Kaplan (1974) on bodily performance in sex was published in this country, it was viewed by the members of the IPM with interest and scientific curiosity, but because of their different findings in the psychosomatic aspects of sex they did not regard it as the 'tablets from on high' as it was sometimes greeted in the communications media. None the less, papers and case studies in the book show that the techniques of Masters & Johnson and of Kaplan have been used with the critical interest that we apply to all our work. The publicity which their work attracted emboldened many who had suffered in isolation to seek help, and men with sexual problems have increasingly presented in the clinics.

This book seeks to give some understanding of the method of training that is promoted by the Institute of Psychosexual Medicine, the findings that have resulted from this training, and the uses to which it can be put. It is not a comprehensive manual for the treatment of sexual difficulties.

Training and Technique

Part I Seminar training

Dr Main's paper was given as the Introductory Address at the Brighton Conference. It forms the keystone of this book, giving the underlying ethos of our work as well as describing the method of training, and its evolution in response to patients' and doctors' demands.

The recording of the demonstration seminar at Brighton was too poor to permit transcription, but I did not want to omit a seminar report as I feel it gives some idea of the non-directive teaching described by Dr Main. Basic seminars are not recorded. The transcript is from Dr Main's research seminar; the doctors have all worked together for some years and feel free to 'speak their minds' though the transcript inevitably fails to give the tones of voice which create the atmosphere. At the time this recording was made the seminar was experimenting with the use of a form on which the clinical material was recorded after an unstructured interview.

1

Training for the acquisition of knowledge or the development of skill?

Tom Main

The prime task of the Institute of Psychosexual Medicine is the training of doctors.

Its method of training requires some eight to 12 doctors to meet at weekly or fortnightly intervals with a trained leader to report to and discuss with each other those ongoing clinical encounters which puzzle them; to give and to get honest comradely criticism about their understanding of not only the patient's conduct but also the doctor's: his characteristic way of responding to the human pain of his patient, and the blind spots, defences and insincerities of the patient and of himself.

The leader does not teach, but requires the doctors to think for themselves. Our training method is in contrast with those intense weekend courses in knowledge which pay no attention to the time requirement for change of the doctor's medical personality.

The training method is investigative of the patient's and doctor's feelings during each clinical encounter. Inevitably each seminar throws up its own findings so that every seminar could be described as one of research-cum-training.

The Institute does not train professionals other than doctors, although the method is of course applicable to other fields of medicine. Moreover it does not require them to be mini-psychiatrists or mini-psychotherapists, but simply to become better at the work they are already doing. They remain body-doctors with some expertise at handling related emotional problems. Sex is something more than a body matter, more than bodily acrobatics: it is also a matter of high passionate feeling and the giving and getting of intense bodily and mental pleasure in the most intimate relationship of all. The sex act is therefore above all psychosomatic and that is why doctors meet the problems they do, for only they have easy access to the body as well as to the mind. Our field of endeavour also distinguishes us from other workers; not just from medical workers involved only in bodily sexual therapy as for the routine treatments of Masters & Johnson, but also from those concerned only with marital relationships or personal emotional disturbances.

The conjugal lives of men and women are complex; the majority of those whose unhappiness is not expressed in psychosexual forms would not dream of going to a psychosexual clinic. People need access to many kinds of help. Thus members of this Institute are trained for a distinct field.

Training for skill rather than knowledge

A doctor embarking on this training should understand the nature of his undertaking; he should be an active practising doctor in the field and prepared to submit his work to critical discussion by co-equals and to comment on the work of his fellows.

Knowledge can be taught — by a scholar to a pupil. Skill must be acquired — by daily practice with efforts to improve it. In the acquisition of skill it is the individual who in the end must decide what to do; for speed of acquisition the individual may find it better to seek the help of a coach who can point out where his practice is going well and where there is room for improvement. The immense importance of knowledge and of teaching, as distinct from skill and coaching, is self-evident, but they alone do not produce skill, let us say, at football. You can be a world authority on football, familiar with the world's literature on its technique and strategies, with knowledge of all the players who have ever lived, and not be able to kick a ball properly. Expert footballers, though none the worse for knowledge, have skill. They did not study but they practised, under the eyes of coaches, played games and then sought and were given critical appraisal of their own play.

Similarly scholarship in psychology does not by itself equip anyone with executive skill for work with people in distress, no matter how much he may wish to help. Nor would more teaching help him. Rather he must meet distressed people, listen and learn from them and then seek regular frequent informed criticism of his efforts by an expert practitioner; and then try again for years, indeed for a lifetime. It is clear, that for the acquisition of skill, whether in football or in the helping of people, the main work is done by the trainee. He must develop these skills from inside himself by altering his ways, sometimes by abandoning old practices and always by devising new ones. All his coach can do is to provide him with critical company on the way. And — it has to be faced — talents vary and are little affected by scholarship. Moreover, while knowledge once acquired is usually permanent, skill may vary from year to year. The maintenance of any skill requires regular practice and regular comments from informed coaches.

Because our members seek to do better work by becoming more skilled, our Institute does not teach theory or give lectures on treatment but appraises the current practices of its trainees. It offers no general accounts of principles or concepts. Rather the trainees are required to learn from their own work with patients and try again. The Institute seminars study living samples of each doctor's ways with specific patients. What happens between seminars is up to the doctor concerned. Responsibility for the patient remains his alone; he is free to do what he can with what he may pick up in the seminar. No attempt is made to supervise him. But with the support of his colleagues and their regular scrutiny of his work he will increase his sensitivity and become more skilled.

8

The doctors of the seminar are all in the same boat so the atmosphere in the seminar is hard-working and purposeful yet friendly, for the work is among equals and nobody tells anybody what to do.

The contrast between the teaching method — the telling method — and the listening and thinking of the training method is obvious. The expert teacher tells his neophytes what he knows and what they should do and he requires obedient pupils to learn. What he teaches will be taken into the intellectual area of the mind. This teaching method is excellent about static facts in the world around us, for instance, about the human body and its organs. Bodily chemicals come in reliable general patterns and knowledge about them can be applied with some confidence to almost every patient with the same illness. But since no human being's distress is the same as that of any other's the doctor faces each time a unique human being for whom general laws are not enough. The problem now is not general ignorance about mankind, but that the doctor is utterly ignorant about *this particular patient.*

In orthodox medicine, the doctor is knowledgeable, the patient is ignorant. His job is to be fairly passive while the doctor does what he wants, examines, investigates, makes the diagnosis and then gives advice. With emotional upset both parties are ignorant. The patient is not passive and the doctor now is not a teacher ('doctor' means 'teacher') but a listener. His relation to his patient is much more one of equality, co-ignorance and co-endeavour. The two set out as partners trying to understand the problems, with the doctor ignorant but willing to understand. He listens and offers his understanding to the patient somewhat tentatively and then observes how his patient uses it. This is a far cry from the practice of body-medicine. Indeed one of our training problems is to help doctors unlearn the medical model whereby the doctor is the expert who ought to know, and replace it with another model of joining with the patient to discuss the problem, to make sense of it. (It will be noted that behavioural therapists' methods are similar to those of the medical model, with an expert instructing a patient.)

Diacritic or synaesthetic perceptiveness
These two approaches — the questioning and telling method and the listening and trying to understand method — use different areas of the mind. The telling method is like science itself in that it is concerned with careful observations of the external world collected by our senses, and by instruments which assist them. The observations are then submitted to the logical areas of the mind and, after their collation, concepts are introduced and general laws are made about various matters in the external world. It should be noted that logical ordering treats the data as dead material for intellectuial manipulation and that because it concerns *things* it contains *no sense of life or living.*

In so far as this 'scientific' method is used to help human distress, it is by definition concerned with fractionated externals (elements of behaviour, symptoms, selected complaints, etc.) and with logical thinking about these. This method not being concerned with the internal world (the *subjective* world of patient and doctor) demands objectivity and ordered logical thought in the observer. The scientific method has yielded enormous fruit for mankind in the understanding of his material world of things, of dead objects — in chemistry, physics, astronomy — and also in the application of this knowledge to engineering, biology, medicine, etc.

Yet, where human passions are concerned, objective science cannot do more than study and wrestle with external signs. It is in no way concerned with the *experience* of passion because that is subjective. Its pursuit of objectivity actually proscribes concern in human subjective experience.

The second approach, the listening method, operates with a different area of the mind, because it concerns different mental processes. Whereas the first classical scientific method fragments the phenomena under study into elements of a size convenient for accurate objective observation, this second method is concerned with total and whole living states — not fragments but alive dynamic fluctuating states which are subjectively felt by whole (psychosomatic) living people. This second method requires, first, the operation of the part of the mind which is not concerned with logic or order, but with *the sense of being alive*; with synaesthetic rather than diacritic perceptiveness. This kind of perceptiveness is vague and subjective. It cannot be demonstrated to others, it cannot be measured or proven by the usual methods of material science; and yet the subject of this synaesthetic perceptiveness is as sure of subjectively perceived facts as any material scientist can be of his scientifically proven facts. To give an example, a man who feels angry at an injustice is as sure of that as he is that the sun is high above him. For him, his anger is a fact but he can only assert it, not prove it or repeat it at the request of others, for it is a subjective truth and not an objective one. It is however at least as important as objective fact — for it is subjective truths of this kind which animate all human activities and responses and relationships and give life its meanings and purposes.

The understanding of subjective phenomena, impossible by the scientific diacritic objective method, needs its own method, one demanding sensitive listening, an awareness that unconscious meanings may lie behind overt communications, deliberate study of subject/investigator relations, including the feelings and impulses of the investigator and — by identification — those of the subject. It requires study of the joint subjective responses to psychosomatic investigations; then the investigator can make a tentative offering to the subject of their understandings of the immediate events in the relationship and observe the effect of this interpretation. In summary, the gathering of data by empathy (synaestheticia) and then the assessment of it by diacritic thought.

This method needs talents different from those required for material science. The word 'sensitivity' gets fairly near but the talents also include thinking and personal sincerity in relation to others. You will notice that it enlists both synaesthetic and diacritic mental processes. We all know this talent and recognise it when we meet it but no one word can describe it; moreover one rarely meets it in high order in those whose main interest is in intellectual achievement.

The part of the mind concerned with the appreciation and assessment of subjective states is not trainable by the intellectual teaching or telling method. It is developed in the individual by the study and control of his subjective responses to human distress; and this may be better done if it is conducted in the presence of sympathetic but tough-thinking fellows who share similar problems and a similar determination to solve them. Such individuals, though rarely characterised by high personal intellectual ambition, usually turn out to be dogged, intelligent, modest people with a passionate interest in human truth.

Our seminars are concerned with distress which neither the patient nor the doctor can easily understand.

Progress of training
As our trainees have learned their medicine — by and large — on the teaching model, they naturally begin by reporting in seminar in the classical medical way — only about the patient and his problem, the family history, the investigations undertaken, the diagnosis and treatment. It may take many weeks to change from reports on patients to reports on clinical events between doctor and patient. But after some months the seminar will be reporting much less about cases and much more about doctoring — feelings, behaviour, defensive tactics, the way their experience with the patient affects them and what this may reveal about the patient's relations with others. Later, seminar members will have begun to study thought and behaviour. As the months pass, the doctors become honest about their limitations, fears, blind spots, impatiences — not only in relation to what they think about the patient but what they feel.

Behavioural treatment appears to be much in line with the medical model. The behavioural therapist knows even before he has met his patient how to proceed and what to assess. His treatment contains the medically traditional mixture of authority, charity and discipline offered to someone who is required to be passive· and who is not encouraged to think and decide what to do but to learn and do what the therapist says. Like medicine, behavioural science concerns fragmented externals — symptoms — and therefore has more in common with material science and biology than with dynamic psychology, which by definition has something to do with the subjective experience of the personal psyche rather than with behaviour. But behavioural science has popular respect, for it is based on quantifiable objective measures — the methods used by material science for the study of dead material — whereas dynamic psychology concerns the unmeasurable subjective experience of living people. This, although vivid and compellingly true for any individual, is non-demonstrable and non-repeatable for outside observers, and non-falsifiable. It therefore cannot appear respectable to scientific philosophers who are not concerned with hermeneutics. *(filósprodakou paske Serepituial / Julésary lorb)*

Problems of identification with teachers and trainers
In the medical model pupils are expected to absorb the teacher's facts eagerly but not very critically. Many obediently swallow up both the knowledge thus imparted and the image of the teacher; they are liable to become mini-teachers. Indeed some do not seek to be doctors at all — but rather to be keen academics who have never for long left their place of schooling for the independent practice of medicine. Massive identification with a teacher is a fairly common and not necessarily unwelcome result of the medical telling model. Our Institute, which seeks skill and sets its face against the force-feeding of its trainees, nonetheless has produced a few instances of similar identification with the trainer — despite our aim that everyone from the first should practise independently, find his own style and develop his own skills in his own unique way. Some degree of identification with the leader and his ideals appears to be inevitable. Certain forceful leaders seem liable to produce little versions of themselves, no matter how hard they try not to. Identification with the

11

trainer may concern not only his career, his knowledge, ideals and habits of study, what he says, what he does, but also what he does not say or do, and how he behaves to the students, etc. The danger of learning by massive identification is that it produces compulsive behaviour and prevents individuals from thinking. When the life of the trainee is dominated by mental images of the teacher, the teacher has become a burden to his pupil, part of a fixed medical conscience. The Institute aims to allow people to be free and to think for themselves; but we have to recognise our failures. A few trainees have remained unwilling to think for themselves but instead will only wonder what their group leader would do in the immediate clinical situation. That kind of doctor, when baffled with a patient, metaphorically reaches out to the bookshelf for 'holy writ' to save him, simply because he does not use his own resources of thought. This turning to the image of the teacher for rescue occurs when the clinical events are particularly puzzling and frightening.

Failure to stick with a problem and think it through occurs because the trainee has the sort of mind which cannot learn except by identification, or because of some flaw in the trainer's method. Some trainers offer models of someone who does not expect to solve every problem, but who is not content to remain ignorant and even when under strain can continue to think for himself. Identification with their model may not give too bad an end result — a doctor who does not expect the impossible from his patients. But a doctor who pursues any model does not listen primarily to his patient but only to his model. Our leaders are not flawless people; this form of training requires rare skill and trainers vary.

Identification can enter different parts of the model — the instructing trainer can be variously a tyrant, a playmate, another useless ally and so forth. If the trainer is a model of letting other people think, then identification with that may not be too bad for the trainee, who then requires his patients to think. If, however, the trainer seeks only a readiness to believe strictly in what he says, the trainee will require that of his patients. The acted behaviour of the trainer — quite apart from the content of the seminar — therefore has important effects. Will the trainee be one who listens and then thinks? Will he be sincerely tolerant? Or only cleverly tolerant?

Focusing on the task

The leaders learn much from their colleagues in training: about patients and syndromes, techniques of interpreting during vaginal examination, the psychological aspects of mechanical and chemical methods of contraception, and about sexual anxieties and fantasies at various ages. But we have come to develop many ideas about training. Here are a few: the seminar should meet at least once a fortnight — better once a week; it should begin with at least twelve members; it should discuss only the treatment of current cases; it should regard reminiscences as a flight from the task; no theory should be taught, no book discussed; attempts to fit elements of the past and present together to make a coherent picture must be seen as a defence against the study of the actual, here-and-now, doctor-patient relation.

Time and again we have confirmed that the study of the doctor-patient relation is the golden road to understanding. Interest in the patient's past history — the classic defence against this — produces a selection of distorted memories and family myths; but like events in the doctor-patient relation, the very selections and

12

distortions can tell us much about the patient's view of himself (a victim, a jealous adult, a masochist, an optimist, etc.)

It is the *unconscious* elements of the past and the unconscious fantasies associated with them which are pathogenic. They cannot be remembered by the patient, only discerned by the doctor listening in the present and alert to the doctor-patient relation. In contrast with organic medicine, the leader has little interest in a 'good history'. Rather he seeks thought about the patient's use of himself in the present interview ('What is he doing and feeling *now?*') and the light which that throws upon his relations with other key figures in his life.

The seminars are less interested in patients than in doctors and in doctoring — doctors' feelings and defences, their flight from awkward to safe topics, their appeasement of smouldering patients, their resort when frustrated to persuasion and reassurance, and so on. The leaders' studies of doctors in action have taught them a great deal about the anxieties of doctoring in limited settings with very limited time.

Each doctor reports to the seminar in his own words and without notes, that is to say, without secondary revision, just as he does with patients. The seminars will require him to think about how the patient got to him, where the motivation came from, how he thinks about his complaint, what sort of person he is, what it is like to be with him, what his manner is, what history, how he treated the doctor, how the doctor treated him, what atmosphere they produced together, what the doctor said and why, what he thought of saying and did not, what his afterthoughts were, who initiated the next appointment. In brief, the doctor is kept at work assessing his synaesthetic experience.

His account is not interrupted, but after he has finished the members are invited to make comment, not so much to the doctor as to each other; the leader speaks, if at all, last. The discussion is an attempt to understand the clinical event but it also reveals the ways in which each doctor tackles clinical problems.

New trainees almost always offer no thoughts but only further questions, and thus they show how they behave with patients. After the questioning doctor has been given full scope, the leader may ask if he is any further forward with his understanding and if he uses the same techniques in his practice. Is it useful here? In such ways the beginner is encouraged to recognise and assess his habitual methods of doctoring.

During discussion of the case the leader will be guided by one principle — to ensure discussion that might eventually throw light on the particular patients. In other words the discussion is about the living patients and not about their *medical conditions*.

The leader also listens for clues about something which is difficult to describe but highly important for the clinical result — namely, the atmosphere which the doctor and patient create together. The same doctor will create different atmospheres with different patients (variously hard-working, tense, apathetic, businesslike, argumentative, heavy, gloomy, collaborative, friendly, intense, rosy, etc.), and in arriving at conclusions about the atmosphere, full attention will be paid to the doctor's unconscious contribution to it and its effect on the patient.

Difficulties in the atmosphere may lead the seminar away from the prime task — the discussion of doctor-patient relations. Some trainees may seek to use the

13

seminar not for learning but for dependence on the leader consultant, and for them the seminar may be a place where they can get a second opinion easily, with others doing their thinking for them. If the leader resorts to solving the cases, rather than to helping the doctors think for themselves, a dependent group will grow and go on for years, happily, but without any change in the doctors, or any increase in skill. Flight from some difficulties in the prime task may turn to other more hidden tasks — perhaps to show the leader that he is useless. The seminar can be used for gladiatorial contests between two doctors who vie with each other in cleverness, while the others subtly encourage them like spectators on a Roman holiday. Indeed all the phenomena of group behaviour may be observed. The leader's job is, by example and occasional interpretations of events that hold up the work, to lead creative thinking. Only after the doctors have got to know each other can they feel free to praise, criticise and argue, and tell the full truth. Then the leader will have no need to intervene. But one last thing: the doctors meet not for social but for professional reasons, i.e. as Dr Smith and Dr Jones. The use of first names would be seen as a flight from professional relations, to be thought about for the light it throws upon the patient-doctor relation now being discussed.

A survey suggests that a refresher course would be welcome for at least some doctors.

Some findings

I cannot refrain from listing some minor findings made in seminars. The way the patient presents should be accepted at face value, not queried, not reformed, not altered. If a couple come together, the doctor should accept this, but work out by listening how it was they came together and not separately. The doctor should not decide *ab initio* to see single people only, or couples only, but should face whatever difficulties the presentation creates. Similarly bringing in a partner, just because a difficulty has arisen, or sending one partner away, is almost always defensive in purpose but not therapeutic in result. Next, physical examination is sometimes used as a defence to avoid or deflect an awkward doctor-patient relation, by the assertion of a threatened doctor-status. Next, becoming doctory, or changing the topic or turning to important-sounding questions, or advice, are all defences against some anxiety which is not understood. Next, pleas for better behaviour are the result of failure to understand what is going on 'I won't be able to help you unless you are able to co-operate' and other methods of telling the patient to stop being the way he is and become the kind of person the doctor would like, are the result of a failure to understand. Advising the patient seems to spring from the need to assert some sort of status amidst the sea of ignorance. To console or reassure the patient is usually the sign that the doctor does not understand and cannot tolerate the patient's distress. Most reassurance seems to mean 'I don't understand what the trouble is with you, but I wish you'd keep quiet. Please stop being so upset, it worries me'. Next, doctors do not become defensive out of bloody-mindedness or stupidity — only because life in the front line is uncomfortable, difficult and at times alarming. No doctor should be expected to produce ideal reactions to a patient minute by minute, but it is important that defences and the anxieties they hide are recognised for what they are. Next, it is perfectly proper to discuss in the group the professional characteristics of the reporting doctor; but discussion of his personal character is both intrusive and irrelevant. The personal ego is not directly involved in professional work and should not be the subject of comment. The professional ego, that part used in professional work on show in the seminar, needs discussion. It is indeed in the professional ego that one seeks limited but definite personality change.

Such change is always painful. No doctor likes to face the fact that the methods he has been using for years may make no sense. But his fellows in the group know about professional pain themselves and will respect his pains of learning. That pain need not be exaggerated. It is the more bearable because the rewards in skill are high. Awareness of the pains will allow a group leader in turn to tolerate certain phenomena. For instance, the doctor who keeps quiet for several weeks and who does not report cases may be having a painful rethink about his entire approach to medicine following some rough handling by his colleagues.

Significant changes in a doctor's attitudes are not usually consolidated until after about 15 to 18 months of the seminars. The work of the previous months may have shown how much there was to say goodbye to. In general the doctors become more at ease clinically, more curious, interested and confident about their capacity to think and work. They can now better stand being ignorant without attempting premature conclusions. They can listen longer, recognise more, not take things at face value, and can interpret with some skill. Some change will have required the abandonment of habits, techniques and defences which were grown in the past to defend against pain. However, at the same time as old habits are given up, new ones are grown, and practised with increasing confidence and freedom, so that a new thoughtful and elastic technique grows.

I should also mention what the seminars do *not* do.

While the professional ego and its activities are discussed, private neuroses are not. The seminar is not a sensitivity-training group, but sensitivity about *real* ongoing cases is sought. Group phenomena are not discussed for their own sake as they would be in group therapy, but only to throw light upon the case in question. Sometimes the group behaviour actually does this. For instance, a seminar attacked the reporting doctor with comments about her callousness with her patient. The attack was so fierce that the leader felt at one time like protecting the doctor from the group's callousness. The patient had been treated callously by her husband. Her own father still treated her callously. She was ill-treated at work. Now her doctor was callous. The woman seemed to evoke callousness in men. But why were the seminar members callous to this doctor. One member said he had not liked the presentation. The doctor knew she had been awful but had presented her work in a Uriah Heepish way, not like herself at all. She had been cruel and now wanted everyone to like her. What was the patient's manner? Was she a crawler also? The doctor to her surprise suddenly realised that this was so. She cringed and whined. Thus we could see the doctor's identification with her patient. She had felt guilty and had seduced the group to back her up. A group member said they too should feel guilty for not seeing all this earlier and another group member told her that she should stop asking so openly for a beating up! Remembering that the leader had felt like stopping the group's attack, we can see here a series of identifications — with patient, doctor and group (and leader?) all feeling guilty and seeking punishment. Group phenomena of this kind are the stuff of group therapy.

But group therapy has its dangers for it would wipe out the whole purpose of the seminar — the study of doctor-patient relations. Comments about these phenomena are justified so long as they are aimed at throwing light on the patient's plight with her doctor and her home as in this instance.

Participation by the doctors in group discussions is not obligatory, merely available, and most groups are tolerant of doctors who may for weeks on end not contribute very much. Prima donna behaviour is, of course, a different temptation but the group is usually well able to cope with this. Much, much commoner is exaggerated respect for others. 'I have a case but it can wait, and if somebody else would like to present first, that's all right' — meaning, of course, 'I don't want to unless you all give me sanction'. Vying of doctors to present cases is, of course, apparent to all in the group and does not need any interpretation.

The group and the leader will eventually become aware of the different abilities of the doctors, and the different growth-rates. Admiration and envy are often expressed, and 'specialists' at a certain kind of case may be recognised. The doctors learn from each others skills and self-assessment is inevitable. Clever doctors may make the others shy in discussion, slower doctors may induce boredom or impatience. The only solution I know is open discussion of this difficulty and the reporting of this to the director of training, with a request for the doctor concerned to be transferred to a more appropriate seminar.

Our members have treated many thousands of patients and have discussed many hundreds in seminars. They have grown and tested hunches until these have become ideas fit for the more rigorous test of follow-up and some have become near certainties. But the first hunches are grown from clinical experiences and they are not taught. For instance, there is no training in psychoanalytic symbolism, yet certain doctors themselves have noticed that some matters are referred to regularly that they seem to have the fixed unconscious meaning of symbols.

I give one example.

A woman patient whom the doctor was treating for frigidity eventually came smiling and wearing bright new clothes and a new hair-do. In her first session, unkempt and shabby, she had ascribed the failure of her marriage to the filthy basement they lived in. Slime ran down its walls and there was an awful smell of drains; it was cold and dark and she hated to live in it, but there was no alternative. Now, cheerful and kempt, she told the doctor, delightedly, that for the first time they had enjoyed intercourse all week. It was wonderful. Later the doctor asked about the housing problem. 'Oh that's no trouble now, it's great, you see we have had it wall to wall carpeted, and it's as warm as toast. The difference is unbelievable. The smell has gone. We've cleaned the walls, we got new wallpaper and we decorated the kitchen two weeks ago. This week he's worked at night painting the front passage with cream paint. It is really lovely and cosy.' It is not possible to hear this sort of material without noticing that improvement in a woman's attitudes towards the genitals often coincides with an altered attitude towards her housing situation. A symbol for her body. Complaints about sexual unhappiness in newly married couples often coincide with complaints about accommodation. For instance one couple lived with the wife's mother. Intercourse was impossible 'because the walls are thin and mother will hear'. Various doctors have found that this fearful sort of reference to the mother is common in those who cannot enjoy sex without guilt, and that treatment of the sexual guilt in relation to mother may be enough to liberate the patient to enjoy intercourse. But it has several times been observed that after the improvement the patient will write to say 'I'm sorry dcotor, I won't be seeing you again. We are leaving the district, you see we've just got a nice house of our own in X'.

A clinical off-shoot of this new independence from parents after treatment is a new independent attitude towards the doctor. Patients once anxious to discuss their sexual lives may, after achieving freedom to enjoy their sexuality, simply drop the doctor. It seems that sexual unhappiness is something to be complained about to a third party, but sexual happiness is private and the doctor must suddenly mind his own business.

The evolution of the Institute

The prime task of the Institute — the training of doctors — excludes some other tasks. The Institute itself does not offer a treatment service, although all its members work in other treatment settings: family planning clinics, general practice, gynaecological and psychiatric departments, special clinics and so on.

Although rooted in clinical studies and adhering doggedly to its prime task, the Institute has nevertheless grown other secondary functions. It publishes a journal for its members It formally assesses the work of its trainees and grants certificates of competence to those doctors judged by its Assessment Panel to be fit for specialist practice. It holds occasional general scientific meetings for its members. Its correspondence secretary directs patients who seek help to other organisations.

The Institute did not begin with specialists meeting and deciding to gather pupils to teach and spread what they knew. Rather it came into being because a large number of doctors clamoured for training in psychosexual medicine and turned to psychoanalysts who had gathered first around Michael Balint. These doctors were encountering problems they did not understand and sought to improve their insight and skills at handling overt and covert requests for help with psychosexual problems. Balint's seminar began in 1958, my own in 1960, and from 1961 to 1963 several other psychoanalysts completed seminars. But the demand continued to grow all over the British Isles, from doctors already working in the family planning movement but discontented with their skills in treating psychosexual unhappiness. But it was always clear that there would never be many psychoanalysts interested enough to develop training of this kind. Balint held that only psychoanalysts were equipped to do so. I did not agree, and indeed was aware that some very keen psychoanalysts could only teach others to become psychoanalysts in turn. With my colleagues in the family planning movement I wondered if perhaps the trainers in the future could one be drawn from workers in the field. A number of senior doctors were expert in psychosexual medicine, had sufficient understanding of the unconscious and seemed to have a potential for work with small groups. I began a seminar for a handful of selected experienced doctors, potential leaders who cheerfully and bravely set off to conduct seminars outside London. We quickly learned that not all good clinicians would make good group leaders, although good leaders were competent clinicians. These early leaders laboured heavily and at great personal financial sacrifice. A few promising trainees beyond one day's range were flown to seminars in London, assisted by funds put at our disposal by Lady Monckton and administered by Mrs Nancy Raphael, for 25 years the staunchest protagonist of this work in the family planning movement.

First, basic seminars were developed for doctors seeking to increase their skills in their normal work. Then came advanced seminars for doctors seeking to be specialists and work in special clinics; leaders' workshops; and over the years several research seminars have studied new problems as they arose, like vasectomy, requests for abortion, and non-ejaculation.

Our Institute has grown with little financial support from the NHS. It does credit to the enthusiasm of doctors who demanded training skills. It is their Institute, set today to continue its prime task of training. This modest organisation is also the largest training organisation in the world in this field, but our training is an inter-generational matter. We also have the problem that training in skill is slow, highly personal and time-consuming, and it can be offered only to 150 to 200 doctors at any one time. But the best guarantee for the continued life of the Institute is that every generation of doctors will demand a training, because doctors are never satisfied with their skills. In their discontent lies hope for the next generation of patients.

18

2

Transcript of a seminar

Dr L./New Case/Responsible Young Wife

Dr L.   This one was referred to me by a GP who writes: 'This pleasant girl has
          lost all sexual interest in her husband. In the past she had good sexual
          relationships with other partners (she also had a termination of
          pregnancy) and one year ago she had a forceps delivery followed by an
          inverted uterus. Her husband is a good-looking chap, an ex-professional
          footballer with previous sexual experience. She has great affection for
          him but no sexual desires.' So that was how she got to me and she was
          given an appointment at the community family planning clinic which
          was for half-an-hour. The referrer is one I trained in family planning.

Leader   A trainee of yours?

Dr L.   Yes. In she walks. She is a matter-of-fact, controlled, businesslike young
          woman of 27.

Leader   Your relation with the referrer — does he like you or not?

Dr L.   Er — yes, I think so. He came to my seminar for about two appearances
          but took fright very rapidly; now he uses me to refer other patients.

Dr T.   Does he like her or not?

Dr L.   I don't know. Highly mixed I think.

Dr D.   All the trainees send stinking cases, don't they. A spin-off of the training
          seems to be that we get an awful lot of referrals from them but they don't
          come to the seminars very much do they?

Dr L.   He has sent me quite a few referrals and some of them have been possible
          so perhaps we'll forgive him this one. She was a dark, pleasant, ordinary
          girl and I can't remember what she had on at all, it was not remarkable —
          I think a raincoat over a jumper and skirt — nothing oustanding in her
          looks but she was articulate and talked quite easily. Her complaint was
          that she had very little libido and also that she had become much less
          sexually adventurous, it was a much more conventional form of
          intercourse that they were indulging in when they did. What brings the
          patient now? — Oh, *patient's attitude to you?* — businesslike.

Leader   What brings the patient now?

Dr L.   I couldn't answer that question; I can only guess that it's the second
          marriage for the husband and it might be fear of eventual break-up if it
          doesn't get better, although this is in her mind because I don't think the
          husband is really putting that sort of idea forward. I don't really know

why now. *Factual material* is that she is 27, she was married in 1979. Her husband is aged 40. She met him when he was a footballer in Australia where she lived and he then went back to Europe and she moved to Europe and lived with him in P. They lived together for a couple of years and then they got married. Sex was fine in those days, and it sounded as though it was.

LEADER   She would have been aged 20 or so.

DR L.   Yes, then they moved to M. becuase mother owned a retailing business and perhaps because he was getting a bit old for football or because mother needed him...

DR H.   His mother?

DR L.   Yes. They moved to M. and her parents came from Australia and they also live in M. They have one baby aged about two. Her version is that she had a good sex life in P. and the trouble is really dating from when they moved to M.; sex has not been very enjoyable and not so interesting. She immediately embarked upon information about her mother-in-law who was so good, so marvellous and so perfect and liked her so much but in fact she hated her. She didn't say she hated her but that was the message I think, that she couldn't stand this woman. She said 'I have to be a specially good daughter-in-law because my husband's first wife was such a rotten one'. I don't know where that came from, whether that was her husband's expectations or hers. She said 'I get on all right with my husband's two sons by his first marriage, there's no problem there'.

LEADER   They live with them?

DR L.   No, they visit. They live with their mother, I suppose. They would be 19 or 18. They visit this family and she says 'I get on quite all right with them'. Then she criticised her mother-in-law for having a lover and said 'But that doesn't make sense because I lived with my husband before we were married but somehow I can't tolerate that she has a lover'. Of her own parents she said they had moved to be near her and she felt, although she liked to have them there, very guilty that they had altered their way of life; they'd left the two brothers in Australia but somehow she felt guilty and I think also trapped because now the whole family was involved and she said a bit of her wanted to go back to Australia. She said of her parents 'They were so good about the termination. It must have been awful for them but my mother was so understanding and paid for me to come to Europe to have a termination'.

DR S.   P.?

DR L.   That was before she met this man, before they lived together anyway. It wasn't his baby.

DR S.   Oh, I see.

DR L.   Her *concept of self* — she said 'On the surface I seem confident and underneath I am so unsure of myself'. Of other people she sees them as so — this was my understanding of it — 'super and nice'. Nobody she has mentioned is really a human being, they are all super. The *developing doctor-patient relationship* — the atmosphere was businesslike; she was

20

	controlled throughout, talked a lot and didn't really leave me much space to say anything: I was mostly listening. We talked in the woman-to-woman sort of atmosphere. The doctor-patient relationship was egalitarian.
LEADER	In your opinion?
DR L.	Yes., *Interpretations* — I didn't examine her. Somehow it didn't seem to come into it, maybe that came from her I don't know. It was a very non-body sort of consultation, it was all about mind. Interpretations I offered were of her control, how controlled she was with me and how feelings had been controlled. Interpreted to her the hate or conflict about her dislike of her mother-in-law for being so good and also about feeling so responsible for herself, her husband and also that she had a need to look after her mother.
LEADER	Her own mother?
DR L.	Yes. Which in the subsequent interview she elaborated on a bit more. The sexual disturbance is shown by a certain misery, guilt and self-chastisement which stops her having sexual enjoyment. The *meaning in psychodynamic terms* seemed to me to be a pathological need to look after people and to do good for other people and an inability to tolerate any bad feelings in herself; she had to suffer and couldn't allow herself any human weakness. This all translated into guilt. *Suitability for psychosexual treatment* — she was owning the problem and was quite well motivated and verbalised her miseries. *Points against* — I thought were the difficulty with being dependent, and that was really the first interview.
LEADER	How often have you seen her?
DR L.	Twice.
LEADER	Shall we hear the second one?
DR L.	Has anybody got a second form I can just look at?
LEADER	*Initial expectations.*
DR L.	Rather cautious as to whether this girl was capable of much change in my hands. She seemed to have…
LEADER	Could I go back? *Points for* and *points against* I've forgotten.
DR L.	*Points for* therapy — she is capable of understanding interpretation.
LEADER	The evidence was?
DR L.	She is capable of accepting her need for control.
LEADER	And the hating of the mother she responded to?
DR L.	Yes.
DR S.	I thought it was interesting that Dr L. did not put, and I'm sure it's significant that she had forgotten, that she knew how to do it before. She was sexy before.
LEADER	It's important not to drift into treatment so let's take it through.
DR L.	Well, she took herself to the doctor.
LEADER	Motivation is personal, she's not being pushed. *Points against.*
DR T.	You said *against* her difficulty in being dependent but I was thinking if we interpret that maybe she'll be dependent.
LEADER	Very good indeed, but meanwhile it's a difficulty against treatment.
DR T.	But it doesn't rule it out.

21

LEADER	It's a *point against*. We must always avoid this wild drifting into treatment. Let's look and hunt for them.
Dr S.	I think *against* is the opposite of what I have just said, that by the end of it doctor and patient had forgotten that she once enjoyed sex and therefore that suggests it is quite deeply entrenched.
LEADER	The social setting is against her. Mother, mother-in-law and first wife.
Dr S.	I would again go along with Dr T., that if that is in fact the cause of the secondary difficulty, then that should be interpreted.
LEADER	Meanwhile the environment is not supporting her. Her husband has gone back to his mother for instance.
Dr H.	Was this precipitated by the disastrous delivery?
Dr L.	She never mentioned the disastrous delivery. If the GP hadn't told me I wouldn't have known.
LEADER	It was disastrous for the GP. Maybe he'll get over it.
Dr H.	Well, I don't know. When did her lack of interest come?
Dr L.	Before the baby.
Dr S.	It sounds as though she came very close to saying 'I came to M. with all this bloody family around me'.
LEADER	That's right. What else is against it?
Dr M.	You talked about her feeling of guilt and I get the feeling of her terrible, terrible wickedness.
LEADER	Yes.
Dr M.	The wickedness I think is associated with when she was a wicked girl. She disapproved very much of her mother-in-law having a lover and commented that she herself had had one but it may be that this is what she was disapproving; we don't know whether she didn't take the man from the first wife.
Dr L.	I don't think she did.
Dr M.	Also how nice her parents had been to her over the abortion, and that was the most awful thing, and they still loved her and still helped her in that awful thing; so maybe she is so so wicked, or has been, that …
LEADER	And wants to be again.
Dr M.	That's when she was sexy.
Dr S.	I think her sexuality became public, that she came to M. for her delicious wicked scene and suddenly became public property, parental property. We don't know but I think this was the way she got it across to Dr L. — wasn't it? — as if she was testing you about what you thought about these things; she wasn't exactly 'want to make something of it?' but it's something like that.
LEADER	I was disappointed with one thing which Dr L. said — 'She is now able to enjoy sex on a lower level' — and that is all she told us! I drew attention to that because plainly she is keeping off these other excitements and this is what you are after. These are things which shouldn't be spoken about, and they are the important things. You robbed us, she robs you, she robs herself.
Dr L.	There was something she mentioned she could no longer do. I think it was probably oral sex but I don't know.

22

LEADER	It's terribly important.
Dr S.	But not allowed to be any more.
LEADER	But still dreamed about.
Dr L.	Yes I think you have something, that the previous excitements got rather lost.
Dr M.	But in a way she expiated for this awful wickedness by this caring, good mother — such a splendid mother to these boys. She's really trying.
LEADER	The wickedness has got lost. It's tipping her cap to her parents instead of saying 'To hell with them. I'm going to do all sorts of things which they might not approve of'.
Dr S.	It may not have been forgotten but it can't survive in the bosom of the family.
LEADER	That's psychically true but geographically not very important.
Dr S.	He'll be off on his housing list again in a moment!
LEADER	Yes. If you can settle down well in M. you will be cured!
Dr S.	That's right.
Dr L.	She did say she would like to go back to Australia but of course it wouldn't be sensible.
LEADER	There are these horrible older women who might turn into quite nice people, if you can dissolve them in M. The other thing is the first wife. She's stolen him from her. She's in another woman's shoes.
Dr T.	And bed.
Dr S.	And he's quite a bit older.
LEADER	She's 26 and he has sons of 19.
Dr S.	Very naughty.
LEADER	So the other wife must be what? Forty?
Dr L.	Yes. So she has to be this super daughter-in-law.
LEADER	I don't want to say it but it sounds like the Oedipus complex, taking a man away from a woman of 40 when she was 20 and the first wife would have been 35 which is very old.
Dr S.	Makes sense perhaps, do you think, of why it had to be an egalitarian relationship with the doctor?
LEADER	I don't believe it is.
Dr S.	It's difficult for them to remember the naughty things together.
LEADER	Well, when they start talking about the naughty things there will be an egalitarian relationship. You see you get a conventional doctor like this, no imagination; the fantasy is very clear that is what she thinks about you. After all, you are rather dull and staid!
Dr H.	I was trying to work out the doctor-patient relationship while you were reporting and you gave the impression that you must sit there listening because she brought it all out. I didn't get the feeling that you had strong feelings about her.
Dr L.	I think I felt rather confused, it was sort of complicated.
Dr S.	You didn't sound confused, you sounded as though you knew bloody well that she was a sexy angry bit but that somehow was so aware of her control that you weren't able …

Dr H.	To share this.
Leader	Dr L. is always confused and quiet and does nothing. That's just the technique she uses. She doesn't kick her patients around like — well I'm not going to mention.
Dr L.	I hoped I was puzzling with her.
Leader	Yes, that's exactly it. It's not eglitarian though — well, it is in a way. Dr L. is not a clever doctor!
Dr S.	I'm dying to hear what happened next actually.
Dr L.	Well, nothing much.
Dr M.	It may be that Dr L. sensed that this was the right approach: 'Let's go hand in hand together.'
Leader	Dr L. has no choice.
Dr M.	With this patient she must have taken this line which was helping the woman find it for herself. You were not going to explain it. You did say she had a certain amount of insight.
Dr L.	Well, she gave her own interpretations.
Dr S.	Nonsense! It's very clear to me that you interpreted her difficulty in expressing her rage towards her mother-in-law. It all happened after that and yet you skidded over it.
Leader	And it seemed as if there was nothing dramatic or clever about it. What I am against here is that you are approving Dr L.'s technique.
Dr M.	No, I'm not approving, all I'm saying is that it shows that Dr L. realised in this girl …
Leader	Oh yes.
Dr M.	I'm not telling you!
Leader	Agree, we are not quarrelling as I thought we were.
Dr L.	Shall I go on? When she came back she …
Leader	How much later?
Dr L.	A fortnight later. She was much the same sort of controlled girl. I said 'What thoughts have you had since you were here last time?'. She said 'I am getting rather worried about my feelings about my husband'. It didn't quite come as soon as this but it came fairly soon. She had said in the first interview that he was much more free and easy than she was. She worried about things and thought about things deeply but he seemed to take things in a much more superficial way as did his mother, they were alike that way. In the second interview she took up from that bit and said 'I think I almost despise him for his weakness and superficial attitudes and I am a bit frightened about that because he is such a super chap, he's absolutely anything anybody could want'. Then I said 'How is it this triangle between the three of you — your husband, his mother and you?' She said 'He's got much closer to her since he came to M.'. 'They didn't know each other very well before that because mother and father had been separated and the footballer son had been away all these years, but since he had come back to M. they, because of the business or whatever, had formed a much better relationship.
Leader	The mother and he?
Dr L.	Yes. So I said 'This perhaps makes it difficult for you, that you have to

share your husband with his mother'. She then went on again about the mother-in-law, how awful she felt; she said 'I saw her yesterday. Of course she thinks I'm wonderful. She's so nice to me and I feel so awful about it'. Then quite quickly she turned from that to going on about her own mother, about her abortion and she became quite tearful and much more feeling was showing. Then she went on 'I feel so awful because they've left my brothers — not that they mind, they might come over here. I worry so about my mother. Of course they wouldn't have any idea that this is how I feel'. I said 'It seems that you are very much still the daughter and have to look after your mother'. She said 'Yes I do. I feel so responsible for her'. Then from there we went on to... I said 'You seem to be a very independent sort of person. Probably you find it very difficult in the role you are in now, being a patient and being dependent on doctors for help'. She said 'Yes, it is difficult but in fact it's a great help to talk about it'. That's about the end of the second interview. We talked a bit about her overactive conscience and where that might have come from. She said 'It isn't really my parents' expectation, it's somehow in me that I've got to be good and keep up all these standards'. That was the end of two. If I go back to the form — the *outcome* — about what was expected I think. I felt that I enjoyed working with this girl.

LEADER   It's irrelevant. What's happened? What was the outcome?

DR L.   The outcome is that she is going to come back again ...

LEADER   No no. What was done?

DR L.   I suppose I've enabled her to show a little bit of the more dependent side of her, not all that much.

DR H.   I thought she also expressed a lot of fear that she is losing her husband to his mother. Mother has become quite a rival, hasn't she?

DR S.   And she is not alone in that either. There is a wife, her own mother and who else? She's stolen all away from her brother, her husband.

LEADER   Personally I think she has some feeling about this.

DR S.   I think she has some tremendous feelings about this.

LEADER   The outcome I think was she slowly got in touch with some of her annoyance at these women and she saw something about her attachment to her mother and this caring for her probably out of guilt, but still you are on to it and it can still be explored and the dislike of her mother-in-law, she was able to put it into words.

DR S.   And see that it's at least partly, this morality, from within herself.

LEADER   And her mother's terribly nice to her and she can't voice her discontent at the doctor — I mean at the mother! You didn't pick up this discontent with the doctor either. This was not achieved but the other thing was. You didn't let her see that she was bound to have some thoughts about you even though you may be angelic. It didn't open that gate. The outcome, I thought, was that you were in the foothills of aggression.

DR M.   I wondered too if she wasn't feeling aggressive towards her own mother because her mother has put her in an awkward position; she's feeling rotten because mother has had to leave these two boys behind.

25

LEADER	Mother was so good about the abortion.
DR. M.	People are so good you have an obligation to them.
DR H.	She's trying to escape from mother again.
LEADER	And mother-in-law is simply wonderful — I hate her! This came out in your own way.
DR H.	Also she's trying to enact some sort of physical escape back to Australia, isn't she?
DR L.	She knows that's a fantasy really.
DR S.	What would be even better if she could say to them all 'Go away, I want him to myself!'
LEADER	'And this weak bastard I married who is clinging around my mother-in-law.'
DR S.	It's interesting; I didn't hear that that way — I heard 'These sexual people are to be despised and I'm worried about that'. Mother with her lover and he with his happy-go-luckiness are to be despised.
LEADER	I thought it was his weakness.
DR S.	Oh, I see.
LEADER	I don't know.
DR S.	Perhaps I'm wrong.
DR L.	It was probably the weakness.
LEADER	Not standing up to people.
DR L.	Yes, she ran things at home.
DR S.	What I was getting at is if she despises now punitively the happy-go-lucky bit of herself that used to be there ... I don't know, perhaps I'm wrong about that. Happy-go-lucky people who take it where they can find it is a weakness.
LEADER	She's been very wicked in the past, had all sorts of sexual enjoyments and very odd things, non-kosher sex, holdings hands or something. There's the abortion, there's the living with a man for two years, taking another woman's husband, being daring and now she's going to settle down and be sensible, have a civilised family life. Oh God!
DR M.	She's angry with her husband because he doesn't share this sort of guiltiness, he really doesn't see what she's on about.
LEADER	He likes to be a mother's boy.
DR M.	And she's angry with him because in a way they could enjoy the wicked bit at the beginning but he's not interested now in that way.
LEADER	He has come back to his mother. She has a baby and feels he's gone back to his mother and she has lost this exciting man. What's the name of her lover — the one she has in mind? There are hints there that she is thinking of it or something.
DR S.	The other thing which occurred to me was that her mother ought to have punished her for her abortion and she didn't and somebody has got to.
DR L.	Yes, mother paid for it.
DR S.	That's right, so she's doing that herself a bit, isn't she — I think.
LEADER	I think she's very nice to Dr L. because Dr L. is very nice to her and I think Dr L. being very nice is a bit of a burden on her.

26

Dr L.	I think of this girl as the Enid Balint syndrome, when she was talking to us at the AGM about the pathological need to look after your mother.
Dr M.	This mother can't be very old.
Dr L	She's got a husband. They're a couple.
Dr H.	I think she's wanting to leave mother again, isn't she, and get away from her?
Dr L.	I think she'd take mother with her, I don't know.
Leader	She does her mother so much damage when she has anything to do with a man.
Dr S.	So the bit of her that wants her mother to go back to Australia can't function really; leave her alone with her wickedness.
Leader	What has the mother come to England for? To be near the daughter. So she has got to look after mum, do as she says.
Dr S.	She feels that she's taken her mother away from her brothers as well; that's the undercurrent — this 'thief business' as you called it. I wonder that she dares take any of your time really.
Dr L.	Oh I think she did apologise.
Leader	Well done, that's very good. 'I'm sorry to be such a nuisance.'
Dr L.	Yes. 'I'm sorry to take up so much of your time.'
Leader	'And how are you feeling? All right?' I think you should take this fantasy up directly with her.
Dr T.	You liked her a bit better the second time, you enjoyed working with her, so what was that about? What was happening? That she was being a bit dependent or grateful or what?
Dr S.	She wept a bit, didn't she?
Dr L.	Yes.
Leader	It might make it worse of course. This thing about damage to this mother, what is this damage to the mother? What harm has she done to her mother?
Dr H.	Deprived her of being a grandmother.
Leader	She's got some feeling of the damage she's done because she had the idea of repairing and the trouble with her repairal wishes is that you can't have them unless you've done some damage first.
Dr T.	We haven't heard about her father, have we. It seems to be the dog that barked in the night.
Dr L.	Yes. She does speak of him, but hardly.
Dr S.	He's here with her?
Dr L.	Yes.
Dr M.	I think the terrible thing she's done to her mother is getting pregnant and having to have a termination and her mother didn't pay due credit to that awful act, her mother forgave her, was loving and forgiving and her mother shouldn't have been.
Leader	She stole the right to motherhood; that's her mother's job, not hers. This is the damage that she did.
Dr S.	And I don't suppose she actually achieved that by oral sex.
Leader	As a result she's wrecked her mother's sexual life, there's only room for one sexual life among the females in the family and she stole it and now she's

	trying to give it back. There she is — younger — how can she? It's a wicked world.
Dr H.	And does this tie up with mother-in-law who also has a sexual life?
Leader	That's the one thing she can't tolerate. That's wicked. Far better to have these sick people around, like Dr L., miserable people.
Dr T.	But she's so envious of the mother-in-law enjoying it, isn't she? It's real envy. But you didn't interpret that.
Dr L.	I didn't interpret the envy, no I didn't.
Dr S.	I think it's difficult for Dr L. because of T.'s leg pulling. We all know what Dr L. is like, very good and very easy for people to talk to about these wicked things and it really is impressively missing with this patient, wasn't it? She's not ready yet to trust Dr L. with that sort of thing.
Leader	She'd be frightened that Dr L.'s misery would be increased to hear about these secret wishes that young people have. She knows quite well that our generation never had anything like this. Sex began about 20 years ago.
Dr M.	The mother-in-law is not being horrible to her. She should be because she broke up her son's first marriage. She's more or less saying 'Surprisingly she's very nice to me'. Really we shouldn't expect her to be nice to her because she's such a bad, wicked girl breaking the first marriage up.
Leader	If she could have a decent row with her mother-in-law she would be free but instead she has to be dutiful, a good girl.
Dr S.	Even the first wife by implication, she gets on so well with the sons, even that has to come out smelling of roses. It's certainly how it came across, all sweetness and light.
Leader	She should really say to her mother-in-law: 'Look you bloody bitch, get your hands off my husband. We're leaving. Stop treating me like a daughter; I'm a woman' — something like that. The essence of this is in the doctor-patient relation. Very much uneasy about 'how dare she', so I think she'll look after you pretty well unless you watch it.
Dr R.	She seemed really to complain more about the women than anything else.
Leader	Yes.
Dr L.	Yes, I need to watch it.
Leader	And how to learn to be free when she is beginning to enjoy life, or are you going to possess her? Nice case, isn't it?
Dr T.	She didn't talk much about her own child. Rather an awful delivery, you said , 'an inverted uterus' …
Dr L.	Yes, she never mentioned it.
Dr T.	Another patient might have gone on about it but not this one. Her own mothering is of no importance.
Dr D.	Perhaps it's just payment.
Dr S.	You wouldn't expect her to have an easy birth.
Dr D.	Or even mention it because it was.
Dr S.	Not quite so simple as to say she has become a daughter again.
Leader	She always has been.
Dr S.	She's gone from being a fairly healthy rebellious daughter to being an obedient daughter.

28

LEADER	And what's she going to do about her husband? Get him to say to his mother 'You go to hell'. Difficult!
DR S.	I wouldn't worry about this mother-in-law except in her own fantasy. Mother-in-law seems to be doing quite well really; she's got her own life.
LEADER	Yes, she doesn't fight with her husband — that's the other thing. Does she fight with him at all about their relationship with the mother?
DR L.	No, I don't think so.
LEADER	Gives him away. The business needed him.
DR H.	It sounds as though it did.
DR T.	Mother owns the business and he's come to run it for her.
DR L.	I don't know who needed it most; the mother or the ageing footballer.
DR S.	That's right. If he's a happy-go-lucky chap he thought 'Oh well, no more fourth division, I'll go and help mother'. But her vision is that he's back in her pocket or something.
DR T.	The parents — they're retired are they? — fancy coming from Australia to live near their daughter. It's bound to be claustrophobic for her, isn't it? Did she express her feelings about that?
DR L.	She said 'I'm very glad that they've come but I feel so guilty'.
DR S.	I can't make head or tail of this. There's no reason to suppose they're very old. What's all this about?
DR T.	I felt that the mother couldn't let her daughter have her own nice, sexy life; she had to come and home in on it.
LEADER	Come to help with the grandchildren.
DR M.	And very forgiving.
DR S.	Maybe the mother has sensed a bit more the destructive bit of her daughter that goes off killing off her grandchildren than the daughter does actually. She's got to be kept and contained to see that she doesn't get up to that sort of thing. I don't know. It's a fantasy.
LEADER	The mother has come to this country in order to be near her daughter and of course she's a dutiful girl who says 'I must look after my mother'.
DR L.	She's certainly not in touch with her anger feelings.
LEADER	The important thing is the doctor-patient relation, anger there — if it's not seen there it won't be seen anywhere. It's a handicap again with Dr L.'s technique in that she doesn't make it easy for the patient to come out with the hatred. Watch this space!

Part II Experience of doctors in training and practice

The first three papers in this section were given at a meeting which focused on the experience of training in a seminar. I have followed this with three case studies which illustrate the way in which discussion in the seminar has affected the doctor's subsequent interaction with a patient.

During seminar training a doctor will become aware of his own feelings in order to understand the contribution they make to the doctor-patient relationship; the last two papers discuss doctors' feelings of anxiety and vulnerability.

3

Learning experience in a basic seminar

Mary Rees and June Betts

The basic seminar group we belong to meets fortnightly with two leaders.

Our reasons for wanting to attend a seminar were more or less the same. The main reason we had in common was our increasing awareness of the great need of many of our patients for psychosexual help, and our own need for help in order that we might help them. The exposure given by the media to psychosexual therapy was also greatly increasing the demand for help. I had been struggling with a non-consummate couple for quite a while and I felt very anxious and frustrated with my inadequacy in dealing with them. When their marriage was finally consummated, I felt that they had given me as much help as I had given them.

Every family planning doctor is aware that many patients do have problems and takes one of two courses — either to ignore the problems or to seek out the cause and help and treat them. All our members, but sadly not all family planning doctors, preferred the second course.

Our preconceived ideas about seminar training had been influenced by colleagues who were already attending seminars. Dr Betts had a brief chat with a doctor who described how the cases were presented and discussed. The doctor had found the discussing and criticising of her cases very traumatic. This is what Dr Betts expected and indeed found when she started our seminar. I also had preconceived ideas, may I say fantasies, about what I expected from my leader and the group. Initially I felt a great frustration — I had expected much more guidance and instruction and had the ill-conceived idea that I would be taught techniques which would turn me into an instant therapist. I was soon enlightened!

Our leader established basic rules emphasising that we should be a democratic group. One of our main rules, which we confess we broke on numerous occasions, is to discuss only the patient presented and never to generalise or introduce similar cases. No two cases are ever identical.

The influence of the leader is bound to be of the greatest importance, especially, I think, in a basic seminar. Our leader has the knack of being a leader without making it obvious; her verbal contribution is minimal and on no occasion has she ever spoken more than any other member. She is able to guide us through our discussions yet it always appears that we are guiding ourselves. Her attitudes to and methods of therapy were to affect us all greatly.

32

I certainly at first longed for more communication from our leader and felt quite annoyed by her resistance to joining in our discussions and to giving us more advice. We gradually realised that this was a deliberate strategy to make us think for ourselves from first principles and to sort out our own ideas. When she could be persuaded to give her opinion on where we were going wrong and what we should do next she was always an enormous help and her advice was both constructive and very relevant to future work with that patient.

Here are just two examples:

Case Studies

I had been seeing a young married girl who had presented with dyspareunia. She had been attending the family planning clinic and taking the pill for three years before I saw her. During this time she had often complained of dyspareunia, loss of libido and vaginal discharge. Nothing had ever been found but no one had ever questioned her or followed anything up. When I started to see her she explained to me that her father had died when she was only 13 and she had never had a boy friend until meeting her husband. She told me that for some reason she distrusted men and was frightened of them letting her down. She hated her husband's sexuality and his penis revolted her. I thought that her problems must stem from her father's death and if I could overcome this she would be all right. However this was not so. Our leader suggested I should look at her feelings about her vagina and her vaginal fantasies. When I did this I found out that she had never touched her own vagina or examined herself and it was only after we had worked through these problems that her feelings towards her husband changed and her dyspareunia disappeared.

The second case involved a young non-consummated couple. The girl professed total ignorance about all sexual matters. They requested information and I spent a long time talking to them about their anatomy and about intercourse. This made no difference to her vaginismus and our leader said 'I'll lay odds that she imagines, despite what you have told her, that she has a barrier across her vagina which has got to be broken through'. When I next saw her and questioned her, she used almost identical words, and since talking about this fear and discussing her vaginal fantasies she has found it possible to examine herself and to allow me to examine her and be quite relaxed about it. However she has not consummated her marriage yet and I am eagerly awaiting the next seminar to get some more valuable advice!

Benefits of seminar work

The very first things we learnt at the seminar were how to relax and communicate with our patients, the relevant questions to ask them and how to present these cases at the seminar.

We learnt to be open with and sensitive to the patient and to analyse our own feelings for her, to be aware of our response and to try to stand back and watch the interactions and the reasons for them. This was quite a new technique for us. As doctors we are trained to diagnose, to treat and cure — what we were now trying to do was to try and help the patient to understand herself and then to help herself.

Another important thing we learned was that the patient would often produce the same emotions in us, for example, anxiety, fear, anger, or guilt, as she did in her partner and we tried to understand why she did this, and if the knowledge could help the patient. One of the group presented a patient who was complaining of loss of libido. The patient had been investigated previously at another clinic, and described to our doctor how the vaginal examination had been a horrifying experience. She managed very successfully to transfer these feelings to our doctor who deferred her own examination, fearing that this would further upset the patient. In fact, she was colluding with her. In discussion of the case the group pointed this out and the doctor became much more aware of how her patient had transferred her anxieties to her. Unfortunately, this patient defaulted after our discussion.

Seminar training enables us to give each other confidence. We have often been very anxious about our ability to help certain patients and at times have almost despaired, but the group has been able to give encouragement and to bolster confidence.

The experience of others in the group has also been of great value. We have been able to enlarge our own clinical experience, albeit only at a second-hand level. We have also benefited greatly from the stimulus of other people's ideas and their different approaches to the same problem. Seen objectively in discussion, our problems have often appeared much clearer.

The importance of the vaginal examination has always been stressed; one cannot start to evaluate or treat before this is done. The usual primary value of a vaginal examination is to exclude gynaecological abnormality. Again we have had to adapt our ideas. In our work the value is to assess the reactions and emotions to a finger in the vagina and to use the examination to explore these feelings.

We have presented a large number of very varied cases and our leaders have noticed that even in the early days most cases were relevant to our type of therapy. In deciding whether we can try to treat a problem, we have adhered to Balint's comment: 'Take away the primary problem and if you have otherwise a normal person then you can probably help.' When we failed to recognise our own limitations our patients were usually suffering from some psychiatric illness or had severe social problems.

4

Learning in an advanced seminar

(i)

Jane Berry

I found my advanced seminar year a very worthwhile and a very exciting experience: the most changing experience of my whole medical career. So what I am going to say to you is purely a personal interpretation of what happened to me during the year. What was it that made the advanced seminar year and the learning that I got there such a satisfying and changing sort of experience? What actually happened to us all while we were going through this process?

At that time I was a general practitioner working in a very isolated rural area. I did not have a lot of opportunity to see psychosexual cases but what I had noticed was the extreme distress that some patients had, compounded by the fact that I was their doctor living next door to them in their village and they saw me at all the social functions and all the garden fetes. I then started doing a family planning clinic and felt much freer and the patients were more at ease with me in a situation where they would not run into me in the village shop.

So what was it that changed this GP who felt very distressed for the patients and very confused as to how to handle them — how to treat a case of non-consummation — how to stop getting upset and poking a packet of tranquillisers at the lady who wept in the consulting room for so long that my partner said 'What the hell is going on in the waiting room?' I think the biggest freedom I felt in the seminar, particularly in the advanced year, was the freedom of interaction between colleagues. There was no competition or mistrust such as I had found in general practice. This opportunity for total honesty in reporting our patients was refreshing and I found I could share my immense anxieties about these patients with other people who were just as anxious. This was very comforting. Then there was the exciting process of gradually being able to recognise my own feelings about patients and the intuitive feelings that I had had for seven years in general practice; you know when you see Mrs X. in the waiting room, you think 'Oh God, she is coming again'. The seminar gave these feelings a bit of respectability.

Our traditional medical training teaches us to be as remote and objective as we can. So there was all this opportunity for honesty and for interchange of ideas, but my major worry, which lasted all through the first advanced year, was that I did not think we were honest enough. We were too comforting. We knew each other too well and were too ready to jump in and give each other reassurance and comfort. We were not abrasive enough. We had a very experienced leader who sat there and let us find all this out for ourselves. It took me a long time to recognise my own irritation, aggression and, I suppose, over-confidence, and it was not until one very knowing member of the group put me down for the first time that it all became clear.

Another worry I had was this business of second-hand reporting. I was always worried about whether the way I was actually reporting the case to the seminar accurately reflected what had gone on in the consultation. Did this give the seminar a fair chance to help me with the patient? Was I protecting myself, or was I protecting the patient? Mostly I was protecting myself. I was doing things that I dare not possibly tell the seminar about and it took an awful long time to be honest enough to tell the seminar exactly what happened.

I was doing a special session then and getting a lot of men referred to me with premature ejaculation and I got hold of the book by Masters & Johnson (1970) which gave this technique. And for the first 11 patients there was this tremendous euphoria because it did work. But then I got into a terrible muddle with it because the patients kept coming back. Then there were problems with the wives as well, but I still did not have the honesty to go to the seminar and explain this muddle to them.

Certain members of the seminar wanted a didactic system of training where they could just sit and absorb. And they were very irritated because the leader would not give them advice on how they should treat their patients. Then someone pointed out to me that what we were doing in the seminar was increasing our actual skills with the patient as opposed to acquiring knowledge. What we did not know was how to interact with our patients.

(ii)

Dorothy Morgan

It took this little dissertation to make me work out what I had learned in the basic seminar which prepared me for the advanced. I could only think of three things: getting to know myself — surely the most miserable experience and one which I would not want to go through again; a new interpretation and approach to the vaginal examination; and the case history technique. I can only make those three comments and then it all becomes a little woolly because how much does one carry over from the basic seminar?

First, getting to recognise those cases where one can possibly help from those one cannot deal with. Second, the ability to look at one's case load and know that five or seven sessions is quite adequate for some patients; not like in the old days just plodding on and on and waiting for the light. Thirdly, there has been much mention of the use of Masters & Johnson techniques. I must admit that in my very early days I used them a great deal but now very little.

36

I am being deliberately repetitive for whatever the skills of the group leader, the success of the seminar and the advancement of learning must depend on the receptiveness of the individual group member for further learning and good group dynamics to develop within the seminar.

So what have I learnt? In the first place, I would say a change of attitude: that in the counselling situation one comes to grips with the doctor-patient relationship and learns to look at what the patient is doing to the doctor and what the doctor is doing to the patient.

Next, a bringing to terms. In our past experience we have all been in 'doing situations' whether it be in family planning clinics, cytology or child health clinics. We have all been educated in a 'doing situation', making people better. This work has involved a new role for us in that we do not necessarily make people any better but at least we get them to know themselves and couples to know one another and see whether they will accept the situation that they are in.

Third, I would say confidence. In our new training we face overt emotions, but we also learn to pick up concealed emotional tensions such as anger or resentment and we get the confidence to talk the patients through these emotions. Now I am sure you know that when handicapped children are small, parents can cope, but when these children reach physically the same size as their parents problems arise. And they themselves very often prematurely age because of the stresses with which they live. The marital relationship is usually pretty shredded; and parents come to the terrible moment of decision when they can no longer cope with this child in the home. After all these years of sacrifice they are having to accept that the child has to go into an institution. They are very angry, hurt and resentful people. Now without this training I would certainly not have been able to help these people; I will always be grateful for this bit of learning.

Lastly, self-discipline. By this I mean that we all have cases that we like to deal with and those we do not like to deal with. Personally I am always very happy when a patient puts me in a motherly situation. I think what I have learnt during this year is not to allow the wallowing to go on.

5

Insights gained in seminars:
three case studies

(i)

Doreen Anderson

John and Melissa, an attractive couple in their early thirties, came to see me. He was a chef, they had been married for six years and had a three-year-old son. Right from the start Melissa did all the talking and appeared to control the whole interview. She told me how they had watched Dr Bancroft's programme on television, contacted the FPA in London and had been directed to me in Bradford.

She had a pleasing manner and told her story fluently. She said they had never had proper intercourse; their problem was John's difficulty with ejaculation; although he could ejaculate by masturbation, only very rarely could he ejaculate intravaginally. This had been achieved only a few times when she had stimulated him manually and quickly assumed the female superior position. Their son had been conceived this way. She had recently become so fed up that she had had an affair with another man, but she really did love John, she said, and wanted the marriage to work, so they had come to me for help. He sat silently looking very unhappy and saying very little. Her request for help didn't fall on deaf ears and I leapt into action. Although I couldn't help liking this rather bossy girl, I thought I ought to see John on his own without her and, in the meantime, I gave them instructions for sensate focusing and I went home to read up all about retarded ejaculation.

Two weeks later John obediently arrived carrying in his hand a long thin ruler. I knew what I thought it was, but was curious what he considered its purpose was. It was for smoothing over the icing on a cake he was making! He told me he thought the marriage was all right as it was really, and he politely parried all the questions I felt I was being forced to ask, and he gave nothing away. I was left feeling very useless and inadequate and wondering if Melissa was made to feel like this too.

Next time it was the three of us again; I tried to discuss the behavioural approach but she was a bit cross about that. She is an intelligent girl and had already formulated much of this for herself and I realised she was going to feel very disappointed if this was all I had to offer. The interview was again dominated by Melissa who told me of John's strict upbringing, his mother who thought him stupid, his distress at being reprimanded by his policeman father, and how he was set upon and nearly raped by nubile fifteen years olds behind the supermarket — this rich history poured out of her as he sat in silence.

So what did I do next? I called up reinforcements and a male psychologist colleague joined us for the next session. He suggested the contract system of which I had never heard and I was interested to see John come to life at last, as he argued with Melissa about who should clean out the grate and who should wash the dishes.

Alas, at the next interview Melissa came on her own. She said 'John thinks it's a lot of bloody nonsense and is not coming back'. She was very sad and unhappy. I felt awful, and, feeling that she needed comfort and help, asked her if she would like to continue coming on her own, and she readily agreed.

It was now that I started going to the seminar and was able to share my anxieties about this couple. It was noted that she was doing the complaining, not John, and the first thing I had done was to get rid of her and much good that did me! Then somehow I was driven to bring up male reinforcements and only latterly was I getting in touch with this girl's misery. It was mentioned that she might be aware that she was my second choice of patient; however, she was giving me another chance. It was some comfort to know that retarded ejaculators, especially when brought by their wives, are difficult to treat and that the sharing of her pain might be all I could do now.

I went thoughtfully back home.

I had been asked to report back to the seminar and I came back to tell them how much easier it was just to sit and listen to Melissa pouring out all her thoughts and feelings and interpretations. Didn't I think John would make a good homosexual? He seemed so fond of his own body, preferring it to hers; and how she hated the way he left the lavatory door open and didn't pull the chain, and how her mother expected her to be a good Catholic girl and save her marriage — never mind if her husband were a bit kinky. I just sat and nodded now and then, or raised an eyebrow. She seemed to me to be losing some of her bounce and looked drabber and somehow smaller. Reporting this at the seminar it was remarked that though in touch with her sadness, I had not been able to let her express her anger at not being able to say 'Is it all right to want sex for myself?'

Next time she seemed a little happier and told me that John had actually pushed her aside once when packing the car, quite forcibly, although giving her sidelong glances to see how she had taken it. She also told me she had run away from home at 19 and no one seemed to care when she voluntarily returned. She was able to tell me about the sexy dreams she was having and how much she was missing sex. The session after that, she arrived looking radiant. They were having sex, John was ejaculating intravaginally and wasn't it wonderful? They were going to buy a new house and considering having another baby. I was pleased too as I had become really fond of her over this time.

Attending the seminar had enabled me to identify who was the patient wanting help; it let me see that my frenetic over-activity (maybe partly a response to John's attitude) was not rewarding, and the seminar gave me permission to sit quietly, presenting a model of acceptance and calmness which Melissa may have been able to use.

Elaine Cooper

The *presentation* was that of a *problem of impotence.*

The couple were referred by the sympathetic supervisor of the typing pool where Mrs X. was a typist. The supervisor had noted that Mrs X. was very stressed and upset and that this appeared to be due to 'some sort of marital problem'. She and her husband were both 24 years old and had been married for five months.

Their stress arose from their inability to have intercourse due to the husband's poor erection and premature ejaculation. These had been problems before their marriage but they had thought it would be all right when they were married. Mr X. had been to his GP who reassured him, saying 'Don't worry it will be all right'. But Mr X. was still worried. As *always* — reassurance was of *no value.*

Mr X., an engineer, was the youngest of five children. He was, according to both of them, spoilt by his mother.

Mrs X. was an only child. Her father had died of emphysema when she was seven years old. Until her marriage she had lived with her mother in a one-bedroomed flat, sharing a bed with her.

In the discussion Mr X. could not say the word 'masturbate' and the doctor said it for him. He said that he felt uncomfortable and this was difficult for him as sex was not talked about at home.

I examined Mrs X. She was quite relaxed and easy to examine but looked bothered. I commented on this. She said 'I am bothered because I don't know what is going to happen'.

This feeling and fear of not knowing what was going on was reiterated when she said she wanted to attend the next appointment with her husband as she did not want him to feel anything was hidden. She seemed to feel that people hid things from her.

I suggested an active remedy — the squeeze technique.

Seminar reactions

The seminar said I had been 'accepting and optimistic' — a different sort of mother — but also 'instructing and directive', and I was criticised for this.

At the second interview the couple had made some progress and had achieved intercourse on some occasions. Mr X. complained that he felt the need to perform when they entered the bedroom and therefore preferred to make love downstairs. I asked him how he would feel if he was told not to try again until after the next visit and he said he would feel relieved. It was agreed that no intercourse would take place.

Again reporting this interview at the seminar I was criticised for being directive. I saw how unhelpful it was to give this advice and that discussing why he feared performing would have been more constructive.

I tried to see how I came to give this advice and recognised that I was feeling low before the interview as I had returned from my mother's funeral the day before. I was pleased to hear that they had made progress but throughout the interview it was difficult to prevent personal thoughts intruding. I thought I had managed to keep my own feelings hidden. When they talked of their mothers, I thought of mine. They too were having to break the emotional ties with their mothers. It was painful for them too.

When it was discussed at the seminar it seemed that I had kept thinking of my loss because they were thinking of theirs and I had needed to shield all of us from the pain by giving advice. It worried me a lot that I had mishandled the interview.

At the third interview the couple said they were worse. Mr X. said that the advice not to have intercourse had not worked and that they had therefore decided to resume intercourse again and had mutual orgasm. It seemed to have been helpful for him to find that the advice of the 'doctor-mother' figure could be wrong and he had overruled it as he was unable to do with his own smothering mother. He did not like his wife to show her bad feelings and cry — he needed her to be strong. She was afraid that if she showed her feelings he would leave her as her father and previous boy friends had and she would be hurt again. They were, in fact, better and Mrs X. felt that she would come alone for the next session. The uncovering of bad feelings had led to progress just as the group's sharing of the doctor's pain and grief when she reported had brought relief.

Mrs X. came to the next interview in casual clothes. She hung up her jacket as if setting to work. She said she was much better. She seemed to have appraised herself and she was taking responsibility for being the patient. She had set about putting her house in order. She had spoken to her father-in-law and shared with him how he felt at always being put second to his son in his wife's eyes.

Mrs X. had also discussed the marriage problem with her mother who said 'Some men are impotent and have to put up with it'. Mrs X. felt strong enough to put her mother down saying this was not so as they had proved it. She had been angry with her mother and blamed her for their difficulties, saying 'It's because of you I am as I am'. They had cried together and then felt better. I hoped that the mother was not going to be burdened with guilt about this. Discussing this, the group felt that mothers are not so vulnerable.

Mrs X. seemed to be trying to say that she did not need to come any more but was afraid to hurt my feelings. I felt the need to ease her difficulty by asking 'Do you need to come any more?' and when she said 'No', told her that I was very pleased that she could now cope without me.

At the time I did not think to ask why Mrs X. felt bothered about hurting my feelings. At the group later, how to cope with these inevitable pains was discussed and the group's experience indicated that verbalising the difficulty, interpreting it and sharing it was most valuable.

I asked Mrs X. how she would manage if more problems arose and she replied 'We'll face them and talk about them. We've changed about how we feel about bad things haven't we?. I'll come out with it and not stay all silent'.

I asked how it had been when her father died. She said 'I was only seven and he died on Christmas Day. I knew he had been taken to hospital but no one would tell me what was going on. My mother came home and cried and wouldn't tell me. I felt so confused'.

Apparently, from that time onwards she had never verbalised distress. The general feeling in the group was that you need to relive the pain before you can really feel better.

The turning point in this case seemed to be at the interview which I considered to be a bad session, when I was feeling sensitive to feelings about my own mother and her loss. Mrs X. was enabled to work through her bad feelings about the mothers in her life and the loss of her father. She and her husband were then free and able to be adults responsible for, and able to enjoy, their own fulfilling relationship.

<hr>

(iii)

Margaret Gill

Listening to speakers at our Institute meetings over the past two years, I have occasionally tried to imagine what it would be like to be in their place. Terrifying beforehand, I was sure; rewarding in retrospect, perhaps. The one thing I never doubted, however, was that if I were ever asked to present a case it would be a successful one. It comes as a bit of a shock, therefore, to find myself presenting a case which was certainly a failure, and one in which I can only speculate about the cause.

Case Study

The patient was a 26-year-old girl who had been married for six months and who complained that she was unable to consummate because she was too tense. She had been to see a colleague who works in the same family planning clinic as myself. Ostensibly she came for the pill, but having talked about her problem she was referred to me.

Our first interview was short because of a confusion with appointments. The patient, in tears, had persuaded the clinic organiser to telephone me.

The patient was an attractive girl, neatly dressed. She was near to tears but never actually cried, a point the seminar commented on when discussing her very powerful control. The tears were used to make people do what she wanted, it seemed. From the first I found this patient difficult because she made me do all the 'digging', answering in monosyllables or giving the minimum information necessary, then stopping to look at me hopelessly, both waiting for me to take the initiative and yet also somehow challenging me.

My predominant feelings as we talked were of shame and inadequacy. We discussed the fact that she was able to touch herself and use internal tampons but had taken six months to get used to them as they hurt her at first. This and her inability to allow previous boy friends to penetrate her had made her anticipate the problem with her husband.

At the second visit the organiser and I arrived at the same time outside the clinic. As the patient did not seem to be there, I was able to ask the organiser to remind me of the patient's name and notes. I have a fairly good memory but surprisingly I was unable to remember details of this patient, such as how long she had been married or whether she had used internal tampons. You will notice that these were facts elicited by the questioning technique to which I had resorted. When we opened the outer unlocked pair of doors the patient was waiting inside them. I hoped she had not overheard me.

In the second interview I had to work hard to establish any kind of sympathy and I felt I was being unkind to the patient in persuading her to talk. I commented on this and we talked about her problem being a secret she had told no one about apart from the doctor. She said it made her feel ashamed and inadequate, just the feelings I had had in the first interview but had been unable to use at that time. It seemed that both partners were only children who did not communicate easily. I wondered whether they had talked about their difficulty together at all.

When I suggested examination the patient resignedly agreed. She said that she did not fear it but disliked the idea. She was easy to examine with three fingers and had no vaginismus. She was able to say that what she feared was a 'sudden thrust' causing pain, but I was unable to explore her fantasies any further. I was feeling a little warmer towards this patient, and seeing her obvious reluctance to go out through the clinic waiting room I let her out of a side door. When I presented the case, the seminar commented that this patient seemed to think that her secret 'showed' and she was unwilling to identify with the sexual women outside. It was suggested that this might be explored further and that she should come within the normal clinic time.

At the third interview the patient reported 'no change'. She seemed vague about any discussion of her problem with her husband and had assured me before that he would never come to a place like this. She sat looking embarrassed and tearful. I commented on her embarrassment with me and with her husband. I felt like shaking her because of her unresponsiveness. I did say that I found that she controlled me so effectively that I was unable to penetrate her. She admitted that she liked to control things at work also, doing experiments herself so that they were properly done. She said that because her husband did not ask her about our sessions she did not tell him about them. He had never put a finger in her vagina and she had not suggested it. When I asked why, she said that she did not like to do it much herself because it was horrible and slimy. I said that if she felt like that about it, then it was not surprising that she did not want to let her husband in . I suggested she try to talk to her husband and share her feelings with him, something that in retrospect I knew to be very difficult for her.

When I presented this case to our advanced seminar I said that I was stuck. One member said he was surprised, the case seemed to be going quite well and she was able to talk about the slimy vagina at the last visit. Even so I felt impotent with this girl and the seminar noticed that she had conveyed her anxiety to me to an unusual degree.

I put to the seminar my observation that I found myself forgetting material concerning this patient in a way which was unusual. I even had to use my notes in presentation more than usual. What did this mean? Our leader suggested that the feelings aroused in me of being a cruel, even sadistic, doctor were so strong that I had repressed some of them in this way. She was certainly an uncomfortable, even unpleasant, patient to be with at times in spite of her prettiness and her tears. The seminar felt that I wanted to be a nice kind doctor and not a cruel one. We all recognise that the patients we enjoy treating, at least at first, are those who make us feel that we are understanding, sympathetic, intelligent doctors who are of real help to them. If this patient made me feel so cruel that I repressed some of the feelings that she aroused, no wonder her husband had not asked her what was happening or tried harder to put his finger, let alone his penis, into her vagina.

The seminar was pessimistic about the lack of communication with the husband; even though the fantasies of this patient would be worth exploring because they were so difficult to get at, if there was no communication between the couple I might be separating them still further. Had I seen this patient again I might have tried to see her husband if only because she was warning me off so definitely by saying he would never come.

The next appointment was not kept because of a mix-up. I wrote to her, apologising and offering another appointment. She neither came nor rang. I felt very sad and frustrated at this. I had hoped to be able to help this girl and had established, I thought, a relationship of sorts with her. I was well aware of her anxiety and felt that I had been unable to relieve it at all. I was also very curious to know what had gone wrong (or right?). The seminar leader allowed a little speculation, no more.

At a later seminar the question of the pace of treatment was raised. Thinking about it in relation to this case I wondered whether I had been so caught up in the patient's anxiety and apparent lack of progress that I had been too keen to explore feelings and to push the patient, particularly about her husband. This girl may have needed a much more supportive doctor to allow her to talk about her fears and to understand them.

Conclusion

In writing up this case I was forced to think about the ways in which we gain insights from seminars. There are the occasional blinding flashes when something suddenly becomes clear, but more often the process is much more like our work with the patients in that we struggle for understanding, get a glimpse of what is going on from the seminar and go home to worry at the case like a dog with a bone whenever we have a spare moment. Slowly we arrive at some understanding which we can go back and test out with the patient. Here I think we can identify with our patients to some extent. What I have presented is a combination of insight gained in the seminar and what I have made of that as I thought it over. I find that I need to discipline myself to go on working at difficult ideas until they become clearer. Patients, too, find it difficult to go on working at what we have discussed in between visits and so they tend to switch off until the night before the next one. I sympathise with them — it is so much easier but unfortunately less rewarding. I am very grateful to our seminar training for forcing me to think, think, think. Disciplined thinking does not come naturally.

6

Anxiety and technique

Alexandra Tobert

Recently a patient walked in for her third or fourth visit. We looked at each other —
I hoped that I looked welcoming, but I didn't say anything. She grinned and said
'Aren't you going to say "We-ell?"' I was pleased because she is a shy subdued girl,
and even that very gentle bit of cheek felt like progress. I was surprised too, because
I am not aware that I open every meeting with 'We-ell?'. I wondered then — what
kind of doctor does the patient meet? What kind of a doctor does the patient expect
to meet? No doubt expectations cover the whole of the human kaleidoscope and are
based on the patient's hopes and fears and her experience of previous medical
encounters as well as the attitude of her referrer. Some anticipate every sort of
medical activity and cannot believe that 'just talking' can possibly help. Others
who have earlier been questioned and instructed, cut, dilated, sedated, stimulated,
disillusioned, will long to be listened to and understood.

The need to respond to the patient's expectations is one possible source of
anxiety for the doctor. There are, of course, others. The patient's personality offers
always a variant in the equation of relationship providing a challenge for
appropriate response. There is not one personality which is easy and another which
is difficult. The aggressive, the gentle, the erudite and the simple, the extreme and
the mediocre along every human axis may all expose an Achilles heel and thus
undermine confidence. I expect that we are all familiar with the sufferers from the
'mollusc syndrome' whose protective shell deflects all well-meant efforts and who
appear to prefer confrontation to contact.

The setting of a consultation may also make a contribution to the sum total of
anxiety. Particularly in a hospital it sometimes feels as though everywhere
complex, clever, animal, vegetable and mineral remedies are being dispensed,
compared to which our own may seem very abstract indeed. It isn't a far cry from
feeling abstract to feeling inadequate.

We come in time to know our own pattern of panic. Perhaps we talk too much
and, finding it impossible to tolerate a moment's silence, turn the session into a
ding-dong of question and answer; or get busy and advise and instruct or retreat
rather than progress to physical examination or discussion of the past. It seems in
effect to add up to an interference with the growing of a doctor-patient relationship.
We all know that the doctor-patient relationship is above all else the tool of our

45

trade. It is the foundation and the framework of treatment and hopefully of the change that will occur in the patient's difficulties. More doubt and confusion tend to attach to the content of the relationship. Perhaps it is true to say that if the doctor takes good care of the relationship the patient will take care of the content.

And yet — as the stack of filing cabinets grows, the experience which they contain may provide some opportunities for an occasional short-cut. I would like to illustrate this point by a personal view of the treatment of frigidity.

It is often possible to treat primary frigidity by using the insights gained through the doctor-patient relationship. The patient exhibits her feelings about her own femininity by denial or exaggeration; she shows how hard it is for her to be vulnerable, exposed, dependent. An unexpected compliance may indicate an underlying resentment. These and many other patterns of behaviour become available for interpretation which in turn provides the basis of understanding and the opportunity for change.

I think that it is different in cases of secondary frigidity. Here it seems important to explore, often in great detail, the events proceeding and surrounding the onset of symptoms and to give the patient the opportunity of expressing the feelings which are evoked.

It is my impression that just as in some sensitive individuals a second wasp sting produces symptoms much more severe than the first, circumstances occur which awaken echoes of earlier traumata and alter the balance between the sexual drive and its inhibition. The group of patients presenting most frequently are of course those who complain of loss of libido after childbirth. It seems that this is a time when a woman's own experience of being mothered is recalled (not usually on a conscious level) and she may feel again an old unhappiness. Sometimes there is an identification with her own mother, whose sexual life may have seemed to be a sad one. Her own sexual pleasure may then feel rather like eating cream buns in front of a hungry child. Comparable situations arise at any time of life. One patient was a nice cosy woman of 41, a miner's wife, who had fully enjoyed her sexual life until two or three years earlier when she had lost all interest and capacity for pleasure. It was one of those cases where there appears to be no conceivable reason and, beset by anxiety, I chased a shoal of red herrings and finally resorted to questions about her childhood. It was as though I had said 'Open sesame'. Her mother had died when the patient was 14. Her father had remarried soon afterwards and lost all interest in his daughter. We shared the sadness of these memories. Her mother was 38 when she died and her daughter had always feared that she would die at the same age. It was hardly necessary to suggest that although she had not died she had indeed become less alive. She cancelled her second appointment and sent a very happy message. Another patient was one in whom the onset of frigidity coincided with her mother's serious illness and feared death. This was not mentioned spontaneously by the patient and only emerged after a good deal of questioning but, when we began to talk about it, out poured memories of an angry and unhappy childhood. Her return to sexual contentment was rapid.

Although in these and other similar cases, the impetus appears to have come from the eliciting of facts, it is the meaning of these facts in the life of a particular woman, especially in so far as they carry an echo of the past, and her ability to express the feelings evoked, in the context of the doctor-patient relationship, which provide the basis of change.

7

Vulnerability: a case study

Joan R. Coombs

Seminar training accustoms one to the exposure of working with troubled patients and also to the exposure of having one's work scrutinised by colleagues. I do not believe it does anything to relieve the doctor's discomfort and vulnerability; nor should it.

There are two elements to the doctor's vulnerability. The first is part of his own psyche and shared probably by most of mankind. The second element is what the doctor is made to feel in the context of the doctor-patient encounter. Of the doctor's vulnerability only that which is relevant to doctoring will be considered here.

It seems that psychosexual medicine has emerged as a speciality partly because the medical profession has declined to concern itself with matters sexual and with the whole patient. Paradoxically, the task of perceiving the patient as an entity has itself become a speciality.

Many patients come in great fear expecting anything from exercises to hypnotism. Most expect medication. Few expect to talk. They assume that my job is to probe them with accurate, intelligent questions. They think a prescription is the only tangible help a doctor can give and in the face of this belief I feel extremely vulnerable. 'What good can talking do?' they ask.

Case Study

The GP advised the couple to come to the clinic together although the wife had implied that her husband was the patient. She complained to her doctor that she had to initiate their rare episodes of intercourse. They were both attractive, intelligent and articulate. He was rather quiet and shy, she was extremely powerful and fierce, so confident in her control of the situation that I felt alarmed by her and found her difficult to approach. She seemed emotionally isolated.

She told me she had only come to the interview because her doctor had suggested it. She did not regard the problem as being hers. She had brought her husband to be put right and she felt that if it were not for his inadequacy she would be getting enough sexual relief from tension, as she put it.

A truly daunting presentation. Her patronising scorn was not reserved for her husband only as she clearly did not expect me to have stature or authority to deal with her husband's deficiency.

In the face of all this I felt very threatened, inadequate and vulnerable. I felt like explaining my credentials. I wished I had a white coat on or a stethoscope visible. I thought of premature disengagement, a prescription, a referral to an expert, anything!

The story was told entirely by the wife who needed no prompting. It was very much her side of the story and often related with a shocking and callous disregard for her husband's feelings.

They had been married for 20 years and she had never had a climax. She was successful in everything that she attempted but this success had always eluded her. This was because her husband could not turn her on, he didn't understand the rhythms and he could not dance either. She said sexual intercourse was like dancing. I asked feebly if it had anything to do with emotions too but she said again it was more like dancing. She was extremely scornful of him because she had never had an orgasm. She had had previous lovers as a student and was all right with them. Presumably they had not had time to reveal their feet of clay I thought, but dared not say it aloud.

This woman was extremely intolerant of imperfections and vulnerability. She told me she had learned this from her father who had always insisted on her prowess and whom she had always sought to please. Even now she finds herself trying to please her father with her successes.

During this interview she countered every mild observation and interpretation I made as if it were an attack. Her husband spoke very little except to reinforce some of her statements.

I felt that they demonstrated over and over again the maladjustment between them, the defences and the rationalisations and the absence of trusting emotional contact. I also felt therapeutically castrated and offered to see them separately.

I genuinely felt it when I said to her 'It must be awful for you to be so successful in all these things and yet to feel that satisfaction has eluded you'. She may have perceived this as an attack as she declined to see me again, saying she had suffered enough and could not face any more.

Next time the husband came on his own and was much more relaxed. He talked easily. He was an extremely introspective vulnerable man; he was at times tearful as he told me about his feelings. He avoided sexual encounters with his wife because of impotence. During their marrige he had had previous bouts of impotence but even when potent had always felt disappointed after intercourse with his wife; it had always been an ordeal and he always felt as if he had let her down. Apparently neither of them had ever been able to communicate much about their feelings to each other and intercourse had become a trial and a test rather than a safe encounter in which they could afford to be inadequate and vulnerable. It seemed a useful interview in which we were able to discuss varying attitudes to sexuality, emotions and communications. I felt on much better ground.

I suppose one of my anxieties about the male patient is the physical examination as it is always possible that there might be a contributing organic condition. More commonly the patient's anxiety about physical normality can be a contributing factor. I find it easier to examine some men than others.

In this case the emotional maladjustment between the two seemed cause enough for their problem. The question of the physical examination did not arise. To be honest, I would have found it difficult to have examined him.

He clearly found the rambling discussion about sex very reassuring. I was able to mention his wife's vulnerability and defences each time he referred to her hostility. It was easier in the safe setting of the doctor-patient relationship for him to perceive the pain and isolation behind her withering attacks on him. All the time I felt her to be technically 'the patient'.

I regard transference as a natural and sometimes inevitable event in a heterosexual doctor-patient relationship and in some homosexual ones. I believe that if this is understood and confidently handled and limited by the doctor it can be of great therapeutic value, but mishandled it can be a very vulnerable spot for the doctor in psychosexual medicine.

Having at last perceived his wife's vulnerability, the pressing need for trusting warm communication became obvious to him and I hoped that when he was at home unsfported by me he would feel able to allow this.

A month later he returned smiling and much more confident and to a certain extent controlling the interview, which I allowed him to do. Apparently communications between them were much warmer and more tolerant. His wife was much less scornful of him and they had been enjoying themselves far more sexually. He was confident that things would continue to improve. He told me that she had even said his rhythm was better. 'How did you find out about these mysterious rhythms?' I asked. 'She told me', he replied. What an improvement that seemed to represent.

I did not ask him if she had had an orgasm. I was afraid of standardising or belittling the improvement they had made.

It seemed important, as it does with any patient at the stage of disengagement from the doctor, to acknowledge the changes and adjustment that the patients themselves had made. They should not have to be grateful to a third party all their lives however much I might crave some of the credit for this adjustment myself. However, this patient of mine was insisting on reminding me that my patience had helped. I was vulnerable enough to be pleased.

This man certainly perceived my vulnerability in the face of his wife's pain and perhaps saw that vulnerability need not preclude sensitivity and the development of insight and confidence. Did my vulnerability as a doctor make him feel strong?

Conclusion

I believe that vulnerability is inseparable from sensitivity in this area of psychosexual understanding. I worry that invulnerability might be allied to insensitivity. Is vulnerability a sign of weakness? Do we have to always strive for success, strength, power and potency?

For me one of the precious benefits of seminar training is the realisation that, although vulnerable, one can work in a useful way with patients. I have found the courage to see pain, identify defences, both my own and the patients', and to go on working — courage I would not otherwise have had.

Part III Defining the boundaries

The acquisition of any new skill will be followed by an exploration of the extent and limits of its use. The first three papers in this section were all given at a clinical meeting which was 'defining the boundaries' of our work, and comparing it with related disciplines. The merits and limitations of defining the 'patient' as a couple or an individual are examined in the last three papers.

8

Defining the boundaries

Margaret Blair

I have found this a formidable task, because although it is perhaps not too difficult to think 'this is Institute work — that is not', it is much more difficult to think 'why?' and it is necessary to think 'why?' in order to make some attempt at defining the boundaries.

The question could be asked 'Are there any real boundaries, and do we need to define them anyway?' I think the answer to that is that there are limitations and not very clear-cut boundaries, but that if we are claiming for the Institute a special kind of training to do a special kind of work then at this stage of our development we have to try to define what these are.

The Constitution states that our aims are the training of doctors for work in psychosexual medicine through the study of ongoing cases in seminar discussion. Theoretically then our boundaries should be defined in terms of training only but in fact it is not nearly as simple as this. I think the work of the Institute could be illustrated diagramatically by three interlocking circles with hazy edges. The circles would represent training, work with patients, and research. The training is dependent on the work with patients and the quality of the work done depends on the training. Research done in seminars and by individuals leads to an expansion in the fields of work with patients and makes increasing demands on training.

To look at this more closely we have to study the doctors's work with the patients and try to define this first. The original clinical encounters were between doctors in family planning clinics and their women patients who presented them with psychosexual problems while ostensibly coming for contraceptive advice. The patients had thus come deliberately to a place where they could expect that female bodily functions and sexual matters would be discussed. The doctors were untrained to deal with this at first, but in the early seminars they began to look at the tools which they had, i.e. the doctor-patient relationship and the examination of facts and fantasies about the patients' sexuality and female bodily functions.

Through this early seminar training the doctors began to develop skills with these tools, and so, the phrase, 'the use of the vaginal examination' came to have a particular meaning in Institute language. Although all of us here know what we mean by it, it has to be restated now as it has become one of the important differences between our type of therapy and psychotherapy or marriage counselling. When we talk of the psychosomatic vaginal examination we mean combining the ordinary physical examination with an examination of the patient's fantasies and attitude to her own body. These are then used in treatment. But, to make full use of them, the doctor's interpretation and timing have to be right and this is a skill that can only be learned through study of the doctor-patient relationship.

To use the doctor-patient relationship the doctor has to learn to pick up the patient's verbal and non-verbal communications and to build up a picture of her life, behaviour patterns, feelings and defences, and then make some attempt to define the problem. One member of a seminar which I led devised a very useful piece of group jargon — the onion skins which illustrate the way the doctor has to work at the patient's defences, taking them off one at a time and allowing her to acknowledge the underlying anxieties and so get to the hidden feelings which these anxieties are about. This is often done by interpretation, linking together the patient's early difficulties with sexual problems in the present and with the behaviour with the doctor in the interview. It cannot be taught but is a skill that can be developed through our training.

Selection of patients
But there is also the doctor side to the doctor-patient relationship. The doctor has to have some understanding of her own behaviour patterns and blind spots so that these do not interfere with the therapy. She also has to select from the material that the patient presents and decide on a focus for therapy. Selection of patients and choice of a focus is particularly important in Institute work. Here it is perhaps appropriate to talk about the onion again. Many onions, while basically good, have a small area, under not too many layers of skin, which has got to be got rid of. The similarity here is that our patients are almost always persons capable of functioning normally in most areas of everyday life, but there is a small area, presenting as a psychosexual problem, which needs therapy. Patients with whole personality problems requiring long-term weekly or more frequent psychotherapy are not suitable cases for doctors trained by Institute methods alone. To quote from Malan (1979) an interpretation is 'a communication designed to bring out hidden mechanisms involved and therefore have therapeutic effect'. Although in Institute work the doctor makes use of the doctor-patient relationship in this way, the relationship should normally remain superficial and deep-transference relationships should not be allowed to develop. Extensive examination of the unconscious and the interpretation of dreams, as in psychoanalysis, is not undertaken and falls outside the boundaries of Institute work.

The treatment is directed towards making a limited but lasting change in the patient's inner world. It is not normally directed towards manipulation of the environment and the external world but, if it is, that needs to be subjected to the same scrutiny as does interpretive therapy and its rationale understood by both patient and doctor.

Since the early, pre-Institute days, the types of problems presented to the doctors have enlarged considerably, as have the settings in which they work. But, the same criteria can still be applied: (1) Use of the doctor-patient relationship to understand, interpret and modify some behaviour patterns. (2) Use of the psychosomatic examination to elicit bodily attitude and fantasies. (3) Start from or focus on psychosexual problems.

Institute doctors now see not only women presenting psychosexual problems in family planning clinics but antenatal and postnatal patients, those requesting termination of pregnancy, those with gynaecological problems, dyspareunia, discharge, pre- and post-hysterectomy difficulties, sterilisation requests and patients having difficulty with the menopause. They also see those who have, or think they have, contracted VD. Others, seen in general practice, may present even less overtly. Male patients are now seen with ejaculatory or potency problems. Many of these groups of patients have difficulty in the relationship with their own sexual bodily functions or with their relationship to their own masculinity or femininity, and it is this that provides the starting point or focus in Institute work.

The use of the psychosomatic examination to elicit body attitude and fantasies is also relevant to all the categories of patients now included and for this reason the words 'psychosomatic examination' and not 'psychosomatic vaginal examination' have been used.

As already stated, our work is dependent on the use of the doctor-patient relationship to interpret and modify some of the patients' behaviour patterns, but there are some patients, apart from those already mentioned, to whom this cannot be applied and these patients have to be recognised and excluded from this type of treatment and so fall outside our boundaries.

These include:

1. Those patients who are unable to communicate adequately.
2. Some patients from other cultures, particularly when the patient has insufficient language to understand or when he or she is concentrating so hard on the language that the subtleties are missed.
3. Psychotic patients and others who are unable to work with their fantasies as these are so real to them that they are unable to distinguish between fantasy and reality. They are thus unable to relinquish their fantasies.
4. Heavily defended patients who are unable to recognise and make use of interpretation.

But, in suitable cases, in patients motivated for treatment, the particular point about Institute therapy is that the choice of circumscribed focus, often psychosomatic, allows an immediate interaction between the doctor and the patient. In many cases something can be achieved in a few sessions and, while not dealing radically with character problems, enough change may be effected to free the patient to progress.

Training
Although, partly for convenience, we divide our training into basic, advanced and the training of trainers, it is really a continuous process whose boundaries are formed by the limitations of the method and by the qualities of the doctors involved.

The method — regular seminar discussion of ongoing cases — can develop considerable skills in some doctors. But there is a limit to which their insight can be developed by the Institute method of training which is not intended either to be therapy for the doctors or to give them a profound knowledge of their own unconscious, but receptive and sensitive doctors inevitably undergo some change and increase their understanding of themselves. They are thus much better able to understand their own responses to their patients' offers. The doctors must learn to recognise their own behaviour patterns and blind spots which can interfere with and severely limit the therapy. Just as there are patients not suitable for these methods, so there are unsuitable doctors. Amongst these are included:

1. Those who have no feeling for the unconscious or understanding of the feelings of others.
2. Those who have come to the seminar with the wrong expectations and cannot see beyond these, e.g. those who have come only to get help with their own problems and those who have come only to be taught.
3. Those who cannot learn to listen but can only teach or preach.
4. Those whose own neuroses get in the way and cannot be overcome by seminar training.

But those who are able to make full use of the training can learn to:

1. Understand and use therapeutically the psychosomatic physical examination.
2. Build up a picture of the patient's life, relationships and behaviour patterns, be sensitive to the patient's unconscious communications and so use these therapeutically.
3. Select suitable cases for this method of therapy.
4. Make use of the doctor-patient relationship.

And so, by the end of training, some of the doctors can be qualified to treat psychosexual problems by the use of the psychosomatic examination with interpretive psychotherapy using the doctor-patient relationship usually in a one-to-one situation. I have omitted discussion of a one-to-two relationship, i.e. the treatment of couples, although increasing numbers of doctors are now doing this and I think it is within the boundaries of Institute work.

The doctors are not qualified to do group therapy, or psychoanalysis, or to treat the unconscious. Although some work may be done with the interaction between family members, they are not qualified to do family therapy.

Training the trainers. There is another dimension to this as the trainers have to study, again starting with the doctor-patient relationship, some of the group dynamics including the doctor-group relationship and the group-leader relationship.

The work of the leader is to keep the group working, to see what may be preventing it from working and to overcome this; unless the inter-group relationships are understood the leader cannot hope to do this.

Research

Institute research comes out of Institute work with patients, and training. That is, types of problems, method of treatment, whether to see one or both partners, etc., can all be studied in training seminars through honest reporting and frank discussion. The subject matter is therefore extensive and has no definite boundaries but the research is limited by the method of training and the abilities of the participants. Our way of working, which is with feelings rather than with facts and figures, does not lend itself to statistical studies which are easily accepted for publication but a great deal can be done by the study of cases in seminars. It was in this way that in the first seminar in the non-consummation study some of the uses of the psychosomatic vaginal examination were discovered.

Increased research leads us to extend our training and the categories of patients seen, and the link between training, treatment and research continues in expanding circles.

Conclusions
Finally, I think we should return to our objects and aims, which is to be a training organisation for doctors, concerned about the maintenance of standards, and we should not try to create a public image of a 'treating' organisation. That is for individual doctors, or the organisation for which they work. Our efforts should be directed towards the medical profession only, in order to let other doctors know that this form of training exists if they wish to make use of it.

9

The use of Institute technique in marital therapy

Jean Pasmore

What are Institute techniques? I see the Institute's work as firmly rooted in: (1) The use of the doctor-patient relationship; and (2) The exploration of the patient's hopes, fears and fantasies about bodily sensations and symptoms as the usual starting point.

Women patients in earlier years themselves took the first step in starting a doctor-patient relationship by consulting a doctor or nurse concerned with bodies generally and genitals in particular.

Institute doctors now work in many and varied settings and patients present in many different ways, so that it now falls to the doctor to take this step — of relating the patient's presentation to bodily sensations. Sometimes this does not happen until much later in treatment, but the Institute-trained doctor will always be ready to pick up indications of this relationship. In my experience this 'pick-up' always brings a sense of relief to the doctor, bringing the doctor-patient interaction into focus and providing an intimate point of contact with the patient which is immediate and vivid: 'in the here and now' — ' a minor flash' in the language of the Balint Society.

Of these two aspects of Institute work, study of the doctor-patient relationship is not peculiar to the Institute, although it is basic. Such study is important in all dynamic approaches — and, although not always acknowledged, in all behavioural work as well. Rather it is the study of bodily sensations and symptoms, and fantasies about these, on the basis of physical examination, which to my mind constitutes the *unique* contribution of this Institute in the field of psychosexual medicine.

What is marital therapy?

I would define marital therapy as a limited, though not superficial, form of psychotherapy with the aim of helping the partners to enjoy a more rewarding relationship, or of lessening some of the strains and dissatisfactions in the relationship. The second definition is more realistic, and is also a description of the way of working. The dissatisfactions in marriage are due to the discrepancies between the couple's fantasy of what marriage — their partner, or themselves — *should* be, and the reality with which they find themselves confronted. The ways in which patients deal with these strains involve the use of all the 'mechanisms of defence', such as projection, introjection and denial. Therapy has to be aimed first at demolishing these defences; and then at understanding and resolving the underlying conflict which their removal exposes.

The strains in marriage are diverse, but one common theme is mutual anxiety about emotional dependence on the other partner because of fear of rejection, of being let down, or of being taken advantage of, by that partner. These fears may lead to a false independence, which is a denial of the need to depend on anyone. The internal conflict is often seen as if it were a struggle, not in the internal world of each partner, but between the partners. This struggle for power — or, rather, against the need to depend on the other person — invades all areas of the marital relationship — money, work, driving the car, bringing up the children — but shows most clearly in the sexual relationship. This becomes a fight rather than a mutually supportive and enjoyable experience.

The woman expresses her fight with the man by denigrating his sexuality — 'men only want one thing' — and becoming frigid. The man deprives her of satisfaction by impotence or premature ejaculation. Put in common parlance: 'Women won't — Men can't'.

Other types of therapy include family therapy, where the question is: What happens in this family? The approach here is to identify the interaction between the members of the family and demonstrate it to them in the hope that they can modify it. The emphasis is not so much on internal conflicts as on their external expression. In marital work of the kind with which I am familiar the emphasis is on the *internal conflicts* in the partners which, if understood, may be resolved, so lessening the need for their expression in marital strife.

In individual treatment wider issues are considered and more emphasis is placed on the individual's emotional development — past, present and future. For this, work with the unconscious, free association, interpretation of dreams, and explicit work on the transference is needed.

In marital therapy these are only involved in so far as they illuminate the central problem: What happens between these two people?

In the behavioural approach the relief of the immediate symptom is the primary goal.

Selection for marital therapy
    1.   *Excluding unsuitable patients*

        Some patients are unsuitable for any form of dynamic therapy and must be excluded as soon as possible to save them increased distress and the therapist wasted time. This group includes those who are too disturbed, too defended, or unable to use interpretative therapy because of intellectual or cultural difficulties. Usually such people can only be helped by some form of long-term support, which is not available in our settings. However, occasionally, very brief short-term support can be enough to allow the patient to carry on; as with the Pakistani emigrant who was able to take sufficient reassurance from his memsahib therapist to lessen his anxiety about his impotence, although he continued to attribute this to masturbation.

2. *Relation to therapist*

The patient has to be able to engage in a relationship with the therapist and to make use of interpretations, though this by no means implies accepting them wholesale. It does mean, however, that patients can have some hope that help is available, otherwise they will destroy anything good which is offered, to demonstrate that it can't be good enough; like the patient who asks for extra sessions but arrives late for those which are offered.

3. *Focus*

A factor favouring marital work of our kind is the presentation of a psychosexual difficulty in an otherwise healthy person. This allows an early and reasonably circumscribed focus to be identified for treatment and agreed upon between the therapist and the patient.

4. *Motivation*

The most important — indeed, vital — condition for marital therapy is motivation; and it is best when both partners are able to own their own distress over the marital problem and to want help with *that* rather than with individual symptoms. In this respect crisis presentation is often especially favourable, when the distress is acute enough to make the partners seek and accept help against a background of a previously acceptable degree of satisfaction in the relationship.

The impetus to change the marital pattern does not spring only from the individual's dissatisfaction and distress but also from concern for the other partner. This must be distinguished from the false concern so often voiced about the feelings of the partner out of fear, resentment, or as a projection of the sense of failure. True concern implies a recognition of the partner as a separate and different individual. 'I want her to enjoy it, too' is different from 'I am so afraid she will not enjoy it and then she gets in one of her rages with me'.

If these conditions are satisfied they add up to the reasonable possibility that patients may be able to get enough help from intensive work on a narrow focus to free them to develop further on their own. When satisfactory sexual intercourse can be established it seems to have a special value, enabling this development to take place. This is often shown in older patients complaining of non-consummation, who come with a determination to make up for lost time and so are prepared to work very hard on their problem, with surprisingly good results.

I would add a note of warning against those patients who present their problem complicated by too many relatives, thus creating a jungle in which this therapist, at any rate, has found herself frequently lost!

Aims of treatment

Before any work can start, the patient's immediate anxieties must be acknowledged and, to some extent, relieved. These may be about the problem itself, or about the visit to the doctor and what this may entail. Unless these are expressed, the therapeutic alliance cannot proceed. For example, patients sent by hospital or by

GP cannot work until this cause for anger is in the open. This ambivalence towards the therapist derives from earlier unresolved conflicts, often towards parents, where anger and despair have been so overwhelming that normal emotional development cannot progress.

Each partner has to become aware of and able to accept something of their own physical and emotional and psychological natures. For the woman, this means valuing her own femininity rather than seeing it as second-best to being a man; and enjoying the possibilities of her own genitals rather than comparing them unfavourably with the man's — and being open to receive. For the man, it means accepting masculinity — and enjoying his own potency and aggressiveness without too much fear of its becoming destructive.

Problems between partners in marriage can usually be resolved if communication between them does not break down — so restoring this communication is an important therapeutic measure. This involves seeking out the many reasons for failure in communication: guilty secrets, fantasies of the other partner's feelings, and *especially* fear of being thought weak or aggressive by the other partner.

We have to unravel some of the mutual projection systems which are distorting the relationship and impoverishing the individuals. For instance, the woman who is ashamed of her own tender feelings and feels these render her too vulnerable may complain bitterly of her husband' weakness; while the man who fears the power of his own anger will see it only in his wife's rages, and condemn it there.

Techniques of treatment

Settings. In the Marital Unit at the Cassel Hospital the setting *of choice* was joint treatment — for two therapists to see the partners separately, at weekly intervals, for one hour; and for the therapists to discuss their work together between their sessions with the patients. In this setting the problems of each individual had first to be formulated in terms of their own psychopathology. This diagnosis was attempted from the evidence of their present marriage relationship, of their relationship with the therapist, and of their relationship in early life with parents or other significant people. An attempt was then made to put together the diagnoses of the two individuals to explain what happened *between these two people* and how they made use of each other.

Occasionally couples were seen in a foursome, sometimes in the course of joint treatment, or sometimes as an alternative throughout the treatment. In that setting, little attempt was made to relate the difficulties to their historical origins in the emotional development of the partners. Rather, the emphasis was on the immediate situation as demonstration of what happened between them during the sessions. Sometimes this setting did allow communication beteen the partners to be freer. In the safety of the session they were able to own their feelings and to show them to their partner in a way they had been afraid to do before. These feelings may emerge as anger and resentment, but often it is the feelings of tenderness and concern and need which have been concealed.

Sometimes only one partner was seen. This was most useful when the patient had a problem concerned with her fantasies about her own body and its use in intercourse. These difficulties could often be expressed and understood with a woman by making use of the technique of using the moment of vaginal examination to explore her feelings. This technique has been described elsewhere and is especially valuable in cases of non-consummation. Fantasies often expressed are that she is too small for her husband; that the passage is a narrow, rigid tube through which nothing can pass without tearing or splitting; and the very important hymen fantasy, which seems to be a common heritage of all girls and persists in many women in spite of sex education. This was vividly illustrated by a biology teacher whose confidence was eventually won by the doctor, so that during examination she was able to say that she thought there was a skin right across the passage through which her periods had come by 'osmosis'.

When the woman is able to recognise that these infantile fantasies do not correspond with the reality — often when she is able to examine herself — she can then have the confidence to encourge her husband instead of playing into his own fears of damaging her. Many of these marriages are consummated without it being necessary for the husband to be seen as well as the wife. But this approach may only deal with one factor in a complex situation and so may be a preliminary to, or an incident in, joint treatment of the couple.

Focus. In short-term work with the marital relationship it is essential to formulate and keep to a focus. Otherwise the free-ranging associations provide an ever-ready escape route from the pain of discussing the presenting problem.

The *basic* focus is always conerned with the difficulties over masculinity and femininity — the physical, emotional and social roles of man and woman; e.g. a woman who is uncertain of herself *as a woman*, feels inadequate or a failure as wife or mother.

The *immediate* focus deals with defences against this basic problem; and, in this connection, in marital work, must recognise when it is time to stop and allow the patients to 'to use life to grow from'.

Use of the doctor-patient relationship

This is the key tool used in this form of work. The pattern of the patient's relationship with the doctor demonstrates vividly the way in which he or she relates to the marriage partner, and how both of these derive from early relationships in the patient's life. Many of the tensions currently present in the marriage are experienced in the interview between the doctor and patient. Observation of the patient's patterns of relationship and of the therapist's own feelings can be put together and used to help understand the problems in the marriage, but of course this can only happen provided the therapist is able to notice — but not react to — feelings evoked by the patient.

Use of the vaginal examination as an instrument in psychotherapy

The vaginal examination can be used in three ways during marital therapy:
1. Where the examination itself becomes the main focus in the treatment: Mrs C. was a widow, aged 49, whose marriage to an older man had remained unconsummated till his death. She now wished to re-marry but had 'her phobia', preventing any penetration or examination. Her response to my offer to examine her was dramatic — feeling ill, vomiting on my floor and

rushing to the loo — but after 50 minutes she agreed and when, with difficulty, I inserted a finger-tip she was astounded and her attitude changed completely to eagerness. Discussion showed that her stated fear of unbearable pain was really more a fear of rape beyond her control, associated for her with loss of control over her bowel.

2. As an incident in treatment, where it is sometimes done by the therapist responsible for treating the patient, and sometimes by a colleague acting as a technical assistant to the therapist: Mrs E., a nurse in a county hospital, came because of her complaint of dyspareunia. In her treatment with a social worker her many difficulties in relating to her 'playboy' husband became clear. I saw her and examined her, to exclude any organic or psychological problem with her own body. Elimination of these allowed her treatment to proceed, and led to separation from her husband.

3. In many cases vaginal examination is inappropriate, where the focus of the treatment is not on the woman's problems with her own body but on the relationship with her partner. Frigidity is used as a weapon in this battle. This is often so when a woman is frigid with her husband but not with her lover.

This technique — as any other psychotherapy — may lead to uneven development of husband and wife, as in the case of non-consummation where the wife being helped with her fears of penetration highlighted the husband's impotence; and his failure to respond to treatment led eventually to a divorce.

The timing of the examination during treatment depends on many factors, but where the patient presents with an anxiety about penetration it is worthwhile using every effort to get agreement for examination at the first interview as otherwise, if the doctor agrees to postponement, the patient's pre-existing anxieties about the manoeuvre are only reinforced, and she will have a difficult week before the next interview, to which she will come with even stronger defences. Where, as sometimes happens, the patient has presented with problems in other areas of the marriage and after many sessions it becomes evident that there are also difficulties in her relationship with her own body, much depends on the understanding of the previous doctor-patient relationship as to whether examination can be accepted by the patient without it seeming to her an assault.

I have referred here to the use of the vaginal examination which was the prototype of the psychosomatic approach. But the same considerations apply to physical examination both of the male genitals and to some extent to all physical examination of patients, male or female, where many are now using the Institute approach; but the difficulty of using examination of the male highlights the special value of the vaginal examination as a direct entry to the woman's ideas and fantasies about her own body.

I end by stating that there should be no such thing as an 'Institute Technique' — only an 'Institute Attitude of Mind'. This is an attitude of detached eagerness to explore and then evaluate and use all the knowledge that can be derived from experience of the doctor-patient relationship, and indeed from life itself.

10

The Institute and psychoanalysis: debt, differentiation and development

Tom Main

A technique of investigation

What is psychoanalysis? There are three definitions. It is first a technique, not of treatment but of scientific investigation. The psychoanalytic method of investigation requires free associations, listening to all details with no emphasis on any particular utterence but regard for all of them as important, after which the analyst who had listened to all of the facts would make inferences. These would then be put to the test of interpretation offered to the patient. The analyst will observe the patient's response to this.

This method of investigation has scientific rather than therapeutic aims — the investigation of unconscious life. In case this sounds recherché and impossible, let us remind ourselves that every mother makes interpretations. She listens to her baby, doesn't know what it means, but listens long enough and thinks hard and eventually makes a deduction about what it's about, then does something, and then observes whether what she has done is appropriate or not. Thus, she finds out about her baby's anxieties. The psychoanalyst, of course, has the patient's words as well. Be he also listens to the music behind the words and the order in which the words come, what causes distress, what seems easy to say, and so on. That is to say, listening hard is the first part of the technique. The next is to make inferences and the third is to test the validity of those inferences by interpretation.

A body of knowledge

But what about the second definition? Using the technique of investigation certain facts emerge. You have to do something with facts after they have been found; namely, order them into groups, find a general law that can make sense of them, and produce some kind of hypothesis that will embrace everything so far discovered and make sense of the totality. All hypotheses are chancy and need to be confirmed or discarded by later tests. This is so in all science. Hypotheses are not always easy to make, but in so far as they are confirmed by test they also can be ordered and regrouped and made subject to further all-embracing major concepts which may eventually become well-tested theory. Thus a body of knowledge is acquired. The second definition of psychoanalysis concerns this ordering of discovered facts. Psychoanalysis is a body of knowledge about the unconscious, a body of theory, tested, confirmed and retested to explain the facts discovered by the method. This definition is the same as in all science. All science is a body of theoretical knowledge. Freud was a superb clinical observer but not a very passionate theorist. He held findings to be sacred but the theories he devised to explain the facts were not holy for him and he was always ready to discard, revise and refashion concepts and theories in the light of new facts. His writings show his discarding of certain theories, his modification of others and his revolutionary changes every now and then of theoretical viewpoints. Since Freud, psychoanalytical theory has developed enormously owing to the researches of other workers.

The *acceptance* of psychoanalysis as a science is, however, quite different from that accorded the material sciences — let us say atomic physics. The atomic physicist's work is taken for granted. He is an expert who knows a lot about a field which we don't know anything about; and we take his theories for granted and give status without question to him and what he does. The psychoanalylist, however, is not in that position at all. His theories concern the workings of the human mind, and on this matter no one feels ignorant. Everyone, no matter how prejudiced, thinks he knows something, at least about himself and therefore about human minds in general. Everyone grew up to know about childhood — his own childhood — and few will listen to deductions about childhood because his are better and more convincing. To hear 'I'm a bit of a psychologist myself' is common enough: that is to say the layman does not accept amateur status in this field, or the scientific status of the serious worker. So psychoanalysts cannot expect the same degree of goodwill and acceptance and support as atomic physicists. Moreover, Freud's discoveries of the content of the unconscious mind are utterly distasteful to those who prefer beliefs about man's nobility and good intentions to facts about his precarious hold on himself in the face of infantile longings throughout adulthood. Freud's theories followed the new facts and certainly were not simply hunches pulled out of thin air. If any theory is precise enough and tested enough it must be respected for it is all we can ever have in the way of knowledge. But all theory is tentative.

A method of treatment
Back to the definitions. Psychoanalysis is first an investigation, next a body of knowledge and last — and here's the third definition — it is a method of treatment for neurosis. Freud valued this last definition least. He had found out that his method of investigation produced insights not only in the analyst but in the patient and that these had liberating effects on the patient. Freud was not, however, *primarily* concerned with helping patients but with investigation of the area of the mind he had discovered.

The atmosphere in which the investigation is made needs consideration It is not, despite popular belief, that of a cold analyst, tearing credulous people to pieces with painful insights. That would get nowhere, anyhow. Psychoanalysis is a collaborative effort, which eases anxieties not by processes of soothing but by understanding and interpretation of the facts behind suffering. Defences, as well as affects, are unearthed and traced to their origins in a collaborative effort. It is not a 'telling' method, as are admonition, advice, behaviour therapy, persuasion, hypnosis, etc., where the therapist knows what to do. In psychoanalysis it is correctly assumed that the psychoanalyst knows nothing and has to find out. There is no consoling, no reassuring, no advice, no moralising, no judgement, no instructing, simply observation and an attempt to understand — a search for the truth. The truth itself gives trouble, because it is often painful; everyone is aware of features inside himself which he doesn't like and doesn't want other people to know about, and which he doesn't want to face honestly. The truth about unconscious features is even less welcome — they are not unconscious for nothing. The search for truth about unconscious matters can be painful and the analyst needs great care and compassion. He is aware he will get nowhere unless this is so. He has to fashion his interpretations honestly and fully but in ways which disturb the patient optimally, i.e. he has to relieve enough anxiety in the patient for analysis to get going and yet maintain enough for analysis to be kept going. Too little and the work will not be done, too much and it will get frozen.

The psychoanalytical investigation is concerned, however, not simply with what the patient says but with what is going on between the patient and the analyst. Quite early in his work Freud discovered that the patient's feelings, attitudes and memories sometimes related to the analyst himself and he at first regarded this as a nuisance because it stopped him investigating the patient's uninterfered-with mind. However, the presence of the analyst was *always* something the patient was aware of and this awareness affected what the patient chose to say and also stimulated certain feelings in the patient. These feelings were often transferred from relations with past figures and the 'transference', as Freud called it, was eventually realised to be not an interference with the analysis but rather a valuable source of information about the past. From then on Freud began his studies of 'transferred' relations.

The doctor-patient relationship: debt
Psychoanalysts were content with this until it was increasingly realised that the analyst is not just an objective observer but that he too has feelings and that he inevitably alters the situation by exercising these feelings in various ways. For instance the psychoanalyst filled with sympathy, compassion, anger, or boredom cannot help these interfering with his objectivity. Such feelings were then regarded as a second nuisance and the analyst was required to control them by his own efforts and insights. But, in recent years, it has been proven that the analyst's feelings also are a valuable source of information about what the patient arouses in people and how he does it. The psychoanalyst thus deepened his knowledge of various methods of human communication — for example, of the ways a patient can induce feelings even of a kind alien to his psychoanalyst.

The work of members of this Institute is known for its concentration on the doctor-patient relationship. We know that whatever the patient says to us is coloured somehow by our presence, and that what we say and do is somehow coloured by the patient. The total doctor-patient relationship, including the atmosphere built by doctor and patient is, however, something more than the sum of two people's transference and counter-transference. It is a dynamic whole, built mutually, and is inevitable in any human relationship. The words transference and counter-transference are inadequate to describe this. The word 'atmosphere' is vague — but I can't do better, and it means something. If you go into any household for the first time, within a minute you will have picked up an atmosphere about how the people get on — how intense, how bored, how busy, how charitable, how genial, how hard working they are. Each household has its own characteristic atmosphere. Similarly every psychoanalysis, every encounter between any doctor and patient, has its own unique atmosphere, and if each atmosphere is studied adequately it throws a great deal of light on what goes on between the two, and what they do to each other; e.g. how a frustrated patient will make a frustrated doctor behave in characteristic ways which affects treatment which in turn affects his patient and vice versa. At other times the doctor will find himself pitying the patient for having such a brutal husband, and begin feeling angry with a man he's never met; plainly his patient has done something to him and conveyed something to him, not necessarily in words. He may find himself behaving with particular tenderness towards the patient, until he realises that he is attempting to ward off her unconscious charges against *him* that *he* as well as the husband is cruel towards her. Then he may begin to understand what the patient is doing to him.

Similarly in our own work. We know for example that frigid patients make the doctor feel useless and impatient in a frozen atmosphere. We know that an impotent man may make the female doctor concerned and keen to help, and yet that the quality of her compassion may reveal her ultimate scorn for the patient; and that later, if the man remains impotent, her impatience and disappointment may reveal to her the aggressiveness with which he defends himself from women and robs them of satisfaction. The study of what goes on between patient and doctor is common in our work and we know it to be the richest source of information about the patient. We know that the genital disturbance is only part of general disturbance in patients: that impotent men are disappointing, that frigid women are cold, that non-ejaculators give enormous initial hope to their female doctors who then slowly discover that this is all. In brief, in this aspect of our work, we have borrowed from psychoanalysis. Also, as in psychoanalysis, our study of the doctor-patient relationship means that we work with the here and now, with the life of immediate feeling which is being demonstrated before our eyes; we seek to help the patient become aware of the unconscious contributions he or she is making to this relationship *at this very moment*. We also borrow the non-judgemental concern for truth, the technique of listening and trying to understand and make inferences about what is going on, and our awareness that the relationship the patient is forming with us in this immediate moment may contain repetitions of and adaptations to relationships from the patient's past. We use the same ahistoric approach — valuing the patient's history not for its own sake but only in so far as it persists in the present in unconscious ways. We offer our inferences to the patient and then observe the effect of our interventions.

The doctor-patient relationship: differentiation

However, we do not listen in the same way as the psychoanalyst does. He listens to everything, we do not. His treatment is timeless, ours is in a hurry. We select what to listen to and what not to listen to. We interpret at the genital level and we illumine the material in so far as it relates to genital difficulties, but are not expert at

66

offering interpretations of the same material, that might illustrate, for instance, the patient's eating difficulties or capacity for parenthood or work inhibitions. In this we are more in the tradition of general practice than psychoanalysis. The general practitioner examines his patients in no way thoroughly; he does not examine *all* bodily systems before he arrives at a diagnosis. The experienced GP has limited time so examines selectively, or he may make his diagnosis entirely from symptoms and history rather than upon the signs which might be elicited by full examination. Our attention is focused whereas the psychoanalyst's might be described as 'free floating'. We are concerned with the patients' relations to other whole human beings, the relations they have with their own genitals and their partner's genitalia; whereas the psychoanalyst is concerned with the detailed examination of the patient's relations with many other things, e.g. with himself, or infantile relations persisting in the present, with what the psychoanalyst calls 'part objects' — mouth, nipple, faeces, parts of whole people, rather than whole people exclusively. In addition, our patients have selected themselves by seeking help from doctors concerned with psychosexual matters; the psychoanalyst's patients seek help for much wider ranging problems, e.g. obsessions, phobias, depressions, depersonalised states. In brief, our work is narrowly focused and in a narrow field. Apart from psychosexual difficulties our patients are managing their lives fairly well and can work at the doctor's pace. Neither is true in psychoanalysis. We offer the patient little chance of developing and exploring infantile dependencies upon the therapist. By contrast, psychoanalysis — timeless, lengthy and with frequent sessions — provides a setting in which the patient may safely do so in order that these dependencies may be studied and understood. In our work, the principal people in the patient's life are outside the consulting room and we are tangential figures. In psychoanalysis, the therapist may become for long periods the most important figure in the patient's life.

The physical settings are different. The psychoanalyst's rooms, couch and chair and the regular session times do not vary from day to day. The patient's relation with the therapist is exclusive; there is no secretary outside deciding whether the patient should come in alone or with the husband, etc.; there are no other patients around, no busy atmosphere of public clinic or hospital, but much privacy. Our own setting is what the psychoanalyst would call contaminated by outside influences, part of real life, with relatively infrequent sessions and the avoidance of conditions by which the patient may 'own' the therapist and use him in primitive ways for months at a time.

Next, our doctors don't aim to be professional psychotherapists who investigate all and understand all. Although they do some psychotherapy they are also concerned for the patient's body, and unlike the psychoanalyst are prepared to examine the patient's body, particularly the genitalia. Our work concerns us as *doctors* doing *doctoring* and we do not seek only to be psychotherapists. There is a psychotherapeutic *element* of some size to our work, but it may be important for us to remember that wittingly or unwittingly there is a psychotherapeutic element in many relations in ordinary life. The nursing mother who endeavours to understand her baby's needs and respond to them appropriately can be thought of as a psychotherapist. The general practitioner, whether he knows it or so, has psychotherapeutic effects and many practitioners have undertaken seminars, not identical with, but similar to our own to make this element of their work more conscious and deliberate and skilled. Solicitors, particularly divorce court solicitors, attempt their own variety of psychotherapy although few of them are trained. Clergymen, particularly those concerned with mourning, may have some training in the psychotherapeutic element of their pastoral work and so on. Psychotherapy is a general skill, an inevitable part of life, whenever one person tries to understand another. The more training in understanding the better the work may be, but the psychotherapist can lay no claim to exclusivity for his work. The fact that there is a large psychotherapeutic element in doctoring psychosexual complaints is not because we seek to become psychotherapists professionally, but rather that we aim to be better *doctors in this field*.

Psychoanalysis is timeless; there is no time limit and the analyst works at the patient's pace and capacities. In our own work we do not accept patients who are unable to work quickly. This is determined partly by the setting (often an NHS matter) but also by the expectation of patients themselves who seek in a crisis fairly rapid insight without being prepared for major reviews of character formation. They — and we — seek quick but important results and because of this we accept only patients who can work at our rate. If patients can't work at this rate — because of, for instance, severe problems of control, or schizophrenic puzzlements, or phobic reaction formations — then we don't take them on. We are prepared to work only with patients who are keenly motivated, who are in acute pain, and who use words in the same way as the therapist. And we strike the iron when it is hot, at times of crisis.

Training methods: development
Our training methods are not the same as for a psychoanalyst. They are required, during their training, to become familiar with the major literature of psychoanalysis throughout the world, have a vast reading list, attend many lectures on abstract and clinical theory and their historical development. They undergo a lengthy personal psychoanalysis and they practice psychoanalysis under regular individual supervision of their cases. In all this, the teaching relation is one of neophyte and expert. In contrast, our training relationships are between mature practitioners in the field of psychosexual medicine, who seek no major analytical review of their personal lives but rather an increase of their skills in a field in which they are already working; they are not equipping themselves for a different future career, but seek to increase their capacities to cope better with their daily work. The psychoanalyst is required to be knowledgeable, i.e. to have a capacity to conceptualise, or at least to order his work according to existing concepts, and to be able to utilise existing theory in his further researches for truth. Our workers, by contrast, are required only to develop their own clinical sensitivities and powers of observation, and to review, not their personal lives, but their professional lives, geared to a series of existing doctor-patient relationships in daily clinical work. The psychoanalyst might be concerned, for example, with instinct theory or object-related theory, studies of the id or of the super-ego, of primitive ego states, of defensive systems or of psychotic mechanisms. Our own work falls far short of theirs in psychoanalytic erudition and sophistication. But under pressure of clinical facts, our practices contain some details of psychoanalysis. It is clear that our

doctors use the psychoanalytic theory of repression, although many do not know this! In concentrating on the doctor-patient relation they are certainly workers in the theoretical field of object relations and our members' studies in our narrow field seem to me at least as subtle as those of any psychoanalyst in that field. We are aware that unconscious fantasies matter, that tracing distress to its psychic origins is both possible and useful, that Oedipus situation matters, that penis envy is common and yet is defensive, that instruction simply inflates the patient's super-ego and adds burdens to the patient's life rather than freedom: these and many more minor theories of psychoanalysis have been affirmed or discovered by members of our Institute for themselves in work in clinical situations. Our work can justly be described as 'applied psychoanalysis' in the setting of clinics and consulting rooms concerned with psychosexual medicine.

In common with psychoanalysts we do not regard the inculcation of knowledge as a sufficient training for work with people, but whereas the training of a psychoanalyst requries major revisions of his own personality, and alterations in depth, our Institute offers merely the opportunities to change and expand the professional ego, so that the doctor becomes sure and more sensitive about the existence of unconscious distresses in psychosexual matters, and about the efficacy of various responses to this distress. We share the belief of psychoanalysts that knowledge cannot be applied usefully to patients on the couch, but that every patient is a fresh case, which needs its own fresh research. Our doctors and all psychoanalysts share the view that innocence is important and that major data should be collected and put together by the therapist to make good sense before he speaks. The same aims hold true about our trainers — open-mindedness, preparedness to listen, a feel for unconscious material, and the creation of a climate which will allow doctors to review their work in the light of common sense rather than of some morality or professional doctrine.

In yesterday's discussion, the phrase 'hierarchical promotion of ideas' was mentioned and because this concerns a threat to thought, it might be worth underlining it at this point. Those who discover a fresh idea, enjoy it for its explanatory value, and then use the idea as an elastic tool of thought. They can make adventures with it, test the extent of its application, and come to value it. In teaching this idea to others, the delight of the discoverer may at best be felt by his pupils: 'What a good idea, let's try it out.' And they too may enthuse about its freshness and use it as a tool for thought. The third generation having been taught by the second, however, are less likely to do this. The teaching now would be something about the importance of the idea, as if it were a rule, that is 'You ought to remember so and so, it's the right thing to do'. This is far from regarding the idea as something useful, fresh, purposeful. Thus ideas are in danger of becoming empty rules, not a matter for experiment or thought but of obedience and idealisation. In our own field I believe the usefulness of vaginal examination is in danger of becoming hierarchically promoted; from being a useful tip for clinical use, into a rigid rule that it is the thing to do. All fresh discoveries can later degenerate into right-thinking, i.e. into rules, getting 'hierarchically promoted'. The ego is always in danger of being taken over by the super-ego. In this matter we are in the same boat as psychoanalysts. We are in danger once we learn something of becoming sure about it, of losing the fresh ears and eyes, the wonder and innocence of true clinical discoveries — of falling into the trap of becoming experts.

So far I have pointed to our debt to psychoanalysis in the clinical field, and have outlined some of the differences and — at least so far as bodily examination is concerned — some of the developments we have made on our own. But the Institute is not a clinical organisation — it is a training one. It is important, therefore, to recognise that our training method is certainly an application of psychoanalysis to pedagogics, that is to say psychoanalytic knowledge has been used in the devising of a technique in a non-clinical field. Like the psychoanalyst, the trainer does not tell people and does not teach, rather he asks for discussion and continuous case reports, unprepared, unrevised and not containing secondary revisions. He listens to this talk, in much the same way as the psychoanalyst listens to free associations; and then he makes inferences, and communicates these to the group. Like the psychoanalyst he is not there to advise, admonish or teach, but rather to illumine — for instance, by pointing out what has not been mentioned, or how and why the group is defending against its work task (by resort for instance to reminiscence), or he may draw the group's attention to the emotions aroused in it by the problem presented, and how these emotions are being defended, or acted out; that is to say he tries to help the group to think for itself about the clinical problem presented. With increasing experience of this working atmosphere the group will acquire a capacity to discern deeper truths, so that emphasis will eventually shift from discussion about the patient and his problems to a discussion about doctor-patient transactions and, with increasing sensitivity about this, the doctor's skills in investigating suffering and in tolerating distress. Optimally, all will tend to offer their colleagues ideas rather than mere consolation or sympathy or contention. But there is also a limit about what the group does. It does not investigate the whole life of the doctor, but only his professional life. It does not treat the doctor as a person, but only as a professional worker. The blind spots, the predelictions, the prejudices, the evasions and anxieties, which beset *professional* life are open to discussion, whereas the same matters in the doctor's private life are not. As in psychoanalysis, the anxiety level of the seminar is attended to. The complacent seminar is not a very hard-working one; an over-anxious seminar also does not do much work; the aim is a seminar which accepts its difficulties, and yet has the optimism that work can overcome these.

In psychoanalysis the sheer common sense of the analyst, his hard-headed insight, and his tolerance of pain and suffering without resort to frantic defences, offers a model which is, of course, internalised by his patient. Thereby he gains strength in his own ego and becomes more tolerant of and more honest with himself. Similarly, if the seminar group has been dealt with honestly but compassionately the members in turn will become liable to listen to others — colleagues and patients — honestly and compassionately. Our training method is of course a development of that devised by Michael Balint for GPs. It is, so far, the only clear pedagogic method that is an application of psychoanalytic knowledge.

Seminar research
In so far as every psychoanalysis is an individual research, so every seminar is a fresh search for understanding the problems of its doctors. Inevitably discoveries

are made in seminars about the procedures of medicine, about results, about the responses of doctors to various syndromes, about the effects of these responses on patients. Unlike laboratory research, it is not concerned with controlled situations in which a fragment of a problem is selected for study because of its circumscription and its ability to fit in with scientific method. Our own researches deal with uncontrolled situations, but with wholes, not with fragments, whole people eager for help and ready with secrets. There is no possibility of our measuring exactly selected psychological details or of ordering these with complicated statistical manoeuvres into tables and graphs. Our research contains much imprecision but it does tackle major matters. There is however no hope of the seminars producing large series of similar cases undergoing identical treatments for superficial statistical surveys — we undertake fairly thorough studies of unique cases. Thus our researches in seminars yield an utterly different type of knowledge from that which is collected by the methods suitable for material science. We are not concerned to measure exactly the various elements in a series of identically successful intercourses. Rather we are concerned with different experiences of intercourse and the investigation of *unique* living factors which create unique forms of discontent in unique lives.

Allied to the problem of our statistically vague but important research findings, and the impossibility of converting these into the usual graphs which at once both illumine and revivify the practice of medicine, is the difficulty of writing papers about our researches. Writing is the way of reporting deeds and findings, and thus of increasing the world's knowledge. But writing can make little contribution to skills; only practice can do that. The oral method of communication can consider the capacity of unique learners and the pace at which they can acquire skill; and clearly it has its own value. Daughters learn about mothering from experiencing and observing their own mothers; books on mothering, while they have their own importance, do not have the same effect.

In no way do I wish to discourage writing, indeed, I wish to encourage it; but the oral clinical tradition of our Institute is what its training has rested on. Just as the future of psychoanalytical knowledge will be rooted forever in clinical practice, so our writings will concern not conditions nor treatments, nor patients, nor doctors in isolation, but the experiences of doctors working with and being used by distressed people, with studies of relations in unique clinical encounters and the light these may throw on living patients.

71

11

Exploration of the dynamics of seeing couples

'Shall I bring him with me next time, doctor?'

Katharine Draper

Introduction

There have been many dogmatic statements about the relative merits of treating those who present with psychosexual problems as individuals or as couples. Kaplan states: 'It is standard practice in sex therapy to treat couples conjointly' (1974, p. 235), and Masters & Johnson write that 'The marital relationship is the patient, sexual dysfunction is a marital unit problem, never only a husband or wife's personal concern' (1970, pp. 2–3). Those who use behavioural methods (Bancroft & Coles 1976; Begg & Dickerson 1980) offer treatment only when the couple are prepared to attend together.

Within the Institute, where our technique of working was evolved through the study, in seminars, of the doctor-patient relationship in individual consultations, to send for the partner was regarded as an avoidance of pain and stress within that encounter, running away from the focus of anxiety. Now many couples, doubtless due to the reports of conjoint therapy read by both patients and doctors, are coming together to request help, and we must examine our attitude to this presentation.

In this paper I do not intend to add to the dogmatic statements, but to offer you a model that I have found makes a useful framework to stretch out and examine the clinical observations that are made during a joint interview. Furthermore when the entangled interactions are separated in this way I find it easier to understand the pathology, make a provisional diagnosis, and decide on future therapy.

I will go on to discuss couples that I have treated, in terms of the model, and share with you some conclusions I have reached.

The Model

I think of a relationship in terms of interacting wheels; if we do not believe in the static fantasy of 'lived happily ever after', it must be capable of constant movement,

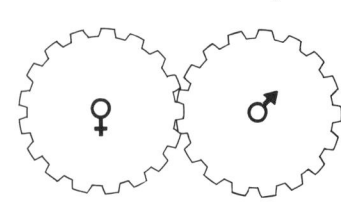

Figure 1

adjustment and adaptation to change. The two wheels represent the man and the woman (Figure 1).

Each wheel, driven from the inner axle, has an outer section representing the face that we present to the world, and an inner core which contains the private world of fantasy, feelings and attitudes that have been moulded in response to each unique experience of development (Figure 2).

Only when the inner and outer parts of the wheel can connect and function together can an individual take part in a sexual relationship, since the drive comes from the inner wheel.

An example of complete failure to connect is seen in a woman who presented with non-consummation, unable to countenance any attempts to penetrate the vagina during intercourse. During therapy she revealed a fantasy about the vagina, that it was a narrow hard tube, with a rigid hymen that would break and bleed, with much pain on first intercourse. Only when this fantasy had been explored — and she had come to understand and accept for herself the reality of her own vagina — could she integrate the inner and outer worlds and progress to a satisfactory relationship (Figure 3).

It is possible to enlarge the model by small wheels, placed at the periphery, which represent factors in the environment that are often blamed for sexual difficulties, e.g. religion, contraceptive use, loss of libido on the pill, work situation, redundancy, post-partum problems (Figure 4).

It is true that difficulty caused by the problem can appear to affect behaviour but further understanding usually reveals that it is not the problem itself, but the way it is used by the patient, i.e. the anxiety in the inner world that is projected in the complaint: e.g., a woman may complain of loss of libido when she has a young baby, blaming tiredness, when the real source of anxiety is her altered feelings about herself and her right to enjoy sexuality now that she is a mother (Figure 5).

For the purpose of this paper the small wheels will be ignored as we wish to examine the interaction in the consulting room.

The two big wheels interact to give the superficial behaviour of the couple, which can be observed during a joint interview. In the microcosm of the consulting room numerous small events show the couple's habitual way of reacting to each other, how they sit, address each other, or me, stay silent, brood, interrupt, try to win favour. For

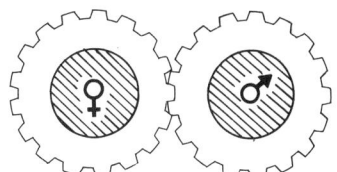

Figure 2

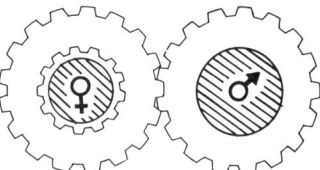

Figure 3

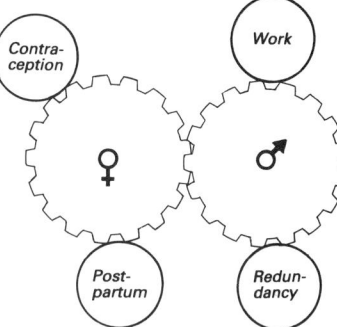

Figure 4

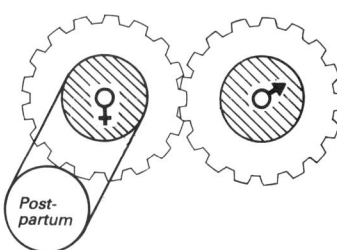

Figure 5

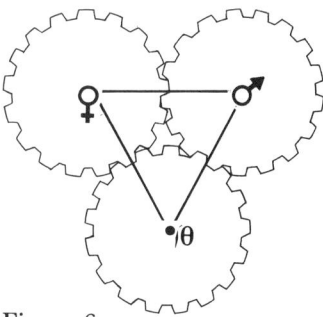

Figure 6

*the moment I will place the therapist in an equilateral
triangle (Figure 6).*

I would like to give an account of the treatment of three couples, and then discuss
my conclusions in terms of the model.

Case Studies

Mr and Mrs A.

The first couple I would like to discuss were referred to the psychosexual problems clinic, by local
consultant physician, with a brief letter stating that 'Mr A. had "secondary infertility" and
increasing lack of satisfactory sexual intercourse for last six-seven years. He was physically healthy
and his external genitalia and prolactin levels were normal'.

An appointment was sent to him, but when I went out to the waiting room I found that they were
both there. As I introduced myself, Mrs A. stood up announcing that as she had taken time off
work to come she might as well come in too. I decided to accept, and examine this presentation. As
they walked into my room I noticed that he, a slim man of medium height, walked with a slight
limp. He sat so that he faced me, but she drew her chair to the side and sat looking at him with a
challenging stare — arms akimbo — one hand on each of her tightly jeaned knees, her spread legs
tapering to smart high heels.

When I asked them to tell me about their difficulty in their own words she just stared at him. In a
depressed soft voice, he said that he had had only very brief erections for the last ten years, and
went on to relate, in a passive way, a terrifying tale of headache, a burst cerebral aneurysm; being
rushed to hospital, his wife being called at midnight to sign for an emergency operation. At this
point she butted in, talking about the fear and anxiety. I noted that she had a marked accent, and
was obviously a more recent immigrant. After months of hospital and two operations he was left
with a hemiplegia, but had now recovered enough to be able to drive and perform all but the finest
movements, and earn a satisfactory living, but 'Sex is different, not so good, and she can't talk
about it — though she's sexy she will never start, and *only* on Saturdays'. She had been sitting
watching this account, a fixed smile on her well made-up face, and I was made to feel sorry for this
gentle, striving but suffering man, and had to resist 'taking his side'.

I turned and started to draw his wife into the conversation. She talked of her job printing betting
slips which meant getting up before six and going to bed early so that on weekdays she was always
too tired, but she said defensively 'I do all I can to help him, I buy "special clothes", dress up and
parade about before him". ('I can't perform to order', he murmured at this point.) As she talked
her face softened and showed pain; and when I said she must feel very desperate at his lack of
response tears came to her eyes.

Then suddenly she shut up, like a clam — 'But you're talking of me — it's his problem — I'm all
right'. When I tried to show her the effect on him of these demands to 'perform' she rebuffed me,
looked upset and reiterated that she was 'OK', going on to hide behind her lack of understanding
English: 'I can't understand what you are saying.'

Asked about their marriage before his illness, I was told that she had had numerous D & Cs
followed by a hysterectomy; these had meant that he had to 'do without it' and she was 'off sex' for
a long time after her hysterectomy. Another revealing fact that slipped out during the interview
was that they never made love when their daughter (now 20) was in the house; but she had recently
married and they felt free to enjoy themselves.

It was time to arrange the next appointment and I thought over evidence that they had given
me. He had shown me by his words, manner and the hurt look in his eyes, that he felt damaged by
his illness and that he was not 'a proper man'; she, beneath her assertion that she was 'fine', and
her brittle, flaunting attempts at sexual titillation had revealed both a deep hurt at his lack of
response and long-standing ambivalence about her own sexuality. There were anxieties in both
their inner worlds, but there was so much to work with in the interactions they had shown during
the interview, which I felt must be resolved before these inner anxieties could be examined. Her
response was that she was too busy and had just come to keep him company, he looked downcast
and hurt. He obviously wanted her to come, and also said, with a hint of aggression, that there was
no financial need for her to work. Finally it was agreed that she would come again.

74

At this point they told me that they had been, the previous year, to the local teaching hospital, and had started behaviour therapy — but it was 'altogether too nosy, and not helpful' and they had stopped going. Just as they were leaving he said that he had good erections at 4 a.m. but she never felt like it then. It was too late for any further work but I felt it showed promise for the future.

Altogether I saw them on three more occasions, at approximately monthly intervals. At first she persisted in her detachment from his problem, and went on to elaborate on her sexy efforts to keep him 'up to mark', and then when interpretations were made, hid behind her poor English — but gradually she came to understand the anxiety created by apparent efforts to encourage him, the way she watched and put him on edge, but always refused when it seemed possible. He was now able to appreciate the pain his failure caused. By examining and interpreting the trivial interactions of the interview there was a change of atmosphere and tension. She was more open and he was more forceful.

At the last interview, early in January, they sat down, both looked giggly, wished me a Happy New Year, and then said that they had 'done it', for the first time for over six months. It was early in the morning but she had encouraged him, and felt marvellous. He expressed satisfaction that he knew it worked and at this point revealed how he had been made anxious by the physician's questions about the hairs on his chest, which generated a hidden fear that something was wrong with his hormones. She talked of her previous difficulty in expressing that she wanted sex, and then fear that sex might precipitate further illness. One of the hospital doctors had told her 'not to let him have it' and they had made love an hour before his aneurysm had burst. This fear was discussed as was a further 'fantasy' — that his father had stopped having sex at the age of 40. He had been able to have a good erection and ejaculation, and he felt better about himself and also valued his wife's feelings of rejection — they had both gained strength by accepting the weaker, softer parts of themselves and each other.

Mr and Mrs B.

Mr and Mrs B. approached the clinic themselves and had made a joint appointment. In their late twenties, and married for a year, Mr B. complained that intercourse was now a rare event although they had been able to enjoy making love while they were engaged. As they sat, facing each other, he said that she had had a series of gynaecological problems, from cystitis to acute dysmenorrhoea. Talking softly and persuasively (he was working with subnormal children) he gave her health as a reason for avoiding intercourse, and when they did make love it was now 'dry' and they used K-Y jelly. She watched him describe her difficulties, her shoulder-length red hair half hiding her well-cut features, and bridled as he recounted her problems. Then she intervened to say that her amenorrhoea on the pill was unimportant as she had never wanted children. She enjoyed her community work and was just starting on a degree, but she had fundamental disagreements on feminist views with James and just shut up — all this was said in a tearful but waspish manner.

They went on to discuss their problems as they saw them. She was illegitimate and her mother had married disastrously, to provide a family; her sister, subnormal, had lived in a home and they were not told of her existence until she died. His father was weak and his mother a bully. I sat on the sidelines unable to use or interpret their self-diagnosis but observing her tearful but aggressive manner and his placating need both to make her the cause of their difficulty and to please her.

This time I thought that there was a great deal of inner anxiety in both, but their clever talk (both worked in counselling others) formed an effective shield which prevented me from being able to.help them. I thought that both were too vulnerable and it would not be appropriate to try and reach their individual anxieties in a joint interview. I suggested separate sessions, on different days, and they readily agreed with this plan.

During first interview she worked through her feelings of being trapped, enclosed, swamped by her marriage; she felt that James wanted total absorption while she wanted space to be herself. Her dysmenorrhorea had only started in the last eight months; the dryness and difficulty occurred when she felt that sex had become a marital duty. Later she reported that they were now discussing and sharing their ideas and he was less resentful of her outside activities and she enjoyed being married. During this time she heard that she had been accepted as a mature student at the university in the town where James was going to teacher training college. She came back once to the clinic three months later and said she was enjoying university life, reading and lectures. All the side-effects she had shown when first on the pill had resolved; she had no cystitis. When they made love she enjoyed it, did not need K-Y jelly, and though less sexually active than when first together she was quite happy with the frequency of intercourse.

When James first came to the clinic alone he talked first of wanting to help his wife but then, after mentioning a couple that was very friendly with, the husband having been influential in his decision to take up teaching, he went on to talk of his own feelings of ambivalence towards his family. Rejecting their bourgeois values he had dropped out from university, lived with a girl friend and taken drugs; he had always felt very lonely at home and his only comfort was masturbation. His weak father was ruled by his mother and he expressed his feelings of fear of 'overtaking' his father, and of showing any aggression — something he demonstrated as he talked to me. One day he arrived late, flustered, he had lost his way (in an area he knew well) but had sufficient insight to see that this was connected with his conflict. He wanted to talk more of his feelings for the friend he had mentioned in the first interview, with whom he maintained an active homosexual relationship. After he had unburdened himself of these feelings we were able to talk of the way he had brought his wife to the clinic, with complaints of her difficulties. Although his immediate reaction was that he would keep coming back to see me from his northern university, after another visit we agreed that he should seek regular therapy locally.

Separate interviews had helped each of them to explore the anxieties of the inner world; Jane had achieved what she felt was a satisfactory relationship, James was happier but still had unresolved inner conflicts, which were now acknowledged and receiving treatment.

I chose these two couples because they illustrate the way in which the insights gained at the first interview can be used to decide upon a course of therapy, but there are times when I find myself defeated by the collusion within a couple.

Mr and Mrs C.

When Mr and Mrs C. first came to see me, he sat with his long, lanky, legs stretched out, his arms folded over his chest, while his wife went on at length about how *she* had taken him to the GP because of his non-ejaculation; *she* had seen he was referred to hospital; *she* had organised his investigation by the hospital doctors. And yet during the interview it transpired that she also refused to use any form of contraception or to consider pregnancy, and was unable to travel to work alone.

Over several interviews I tried to suggest that she might have some fears and anxieties; she became very angry and finally jumped up and marched out of the room. My attempt to explore the anxiety which she was projecting on her husband was felt to be too brutal, and I had completely failed to help them.

Conclusions

When interviewing a couple we start with the couple and the therapist in an equilateral triangle (Figure 7).

But we cannot ignore the fact that the therapist too has an inner world of feelings and attitudes. During a lively discussion, sometimes with a lot of antagonism in the room, it is easy to be drawn to one partner, and this will create distance and hostility or isolation to the other.

The therapist's feelings may shorten the distance to one and create a tension with the other. I was aware that I felt sorry for Mr A. as his wife sat and stared at him, but came to recognise that this was a reflection of the way he felt himself.

I felt the irritation of Mrs B. as her husband paraded her minor gynaecological failings. Without the seminar training I would have felt it difficult not to

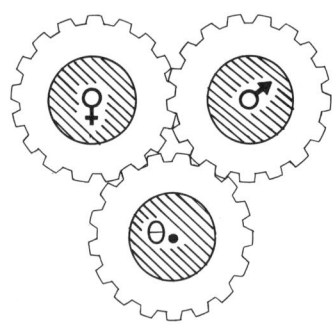

Figure 7

side with one partner, rather than attempt to use these feelings to try and gain insight into their problem.

Our usual work is at the interface between the inner and outer worlds (Figure 8) so that it can be tempting to try and explore the overt anxiety of one partner within a joint interview, but confidences that can be shared and worked through in an individual consultation, as Mr B.'s admission of his homosexual relationship, would be destructive in the presence of the other; work which would be helpful in the one-to-one situation can become very threatening in front of the partner.

If it is felt that there are difficulties in the inner world that cannot be interpreted in the joint interview it is appropriate to see each individual separately (Figure 9).

Whether they are seen by the same or different therapists may depend on availability as well as choice.

If they are seen by two therapists, then consultation between the therapists, perhaps with a supervisor, will be needed.

In behaviour therapy, a co-therapist is introduced to balance the interaction. If we look at this situation, with the interactions of both outer behaviour and the inner worlds I think you will understand why I have not chosen to work in this way. The interactions are too entangled to be used in therapy (Figure 10).

In my experience the most difficult couples are those where there is surprisingly little disharmony, despite considerable sexual difficulty. Here the distorted inner world of one fits with the reciprocal difficulties of the other, and there is strong collusion which can exclude the therapist (Figure 11). The further understanding of these couples is a challenge for the future.

So how do we respond when a patient asks 'Shall I bring him with me next time, doctor?' We can only try to understand what the remark means in terms of the patient who is before us and whether their difficulty is in this relationship or their inner worlds. The joint interview is not something to be 'applied' as a poultice for all sexual problems, it can only be used to interpret and treat difficulties in the relationship; intimate interpretations of the anxieties of either partner are inappropriate.

Like a tightrope walker the therapist must keep his balance, poised between the partners (Figure 12), registering but not reacting to his own feelings, so that he can work with the difficulties in the relationship.

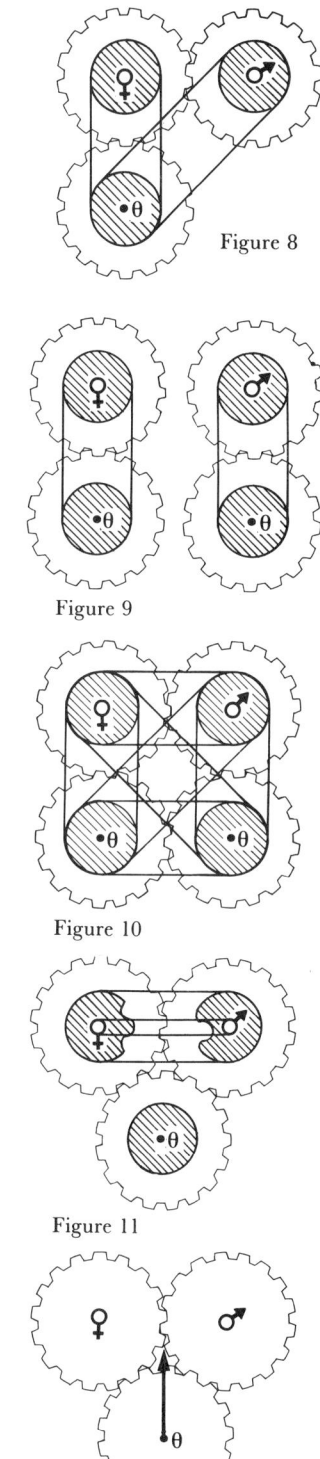

Figure 8

Figure 9

Figure 10

Figure 11

Figure 12

12

Who is the patient?

Ruth Skrine

It has been suggested that I should talk about the hoary old subject of the treatment of couples or individuals — whenever two or three family planning or psychosexual doctors are gathered together, there, within a few minutes, this problem will rear its ugly head. Another suggestion was that we should discuss our own techniques in the face of anxiety in the doctor-patient relationship. I have been aware for some time, as I am sure you have, of the anxiety escape-route offered by deciding to treat someone else—perhaps the partner, or perhaps the couple instead of the individual in front of one; but it was only while preparing this talk that I became fully aware of the alternative escape-route—that is clinging willy-nilly to a well-loved and respectable theory of treatment, often in the face of evidence from the patient that one should be doing something else. The theory can be anything on the continuum from 'In psychosexual work one must always see the couple' to 'In psychosexual work one must always treat the patient who presents'. Is it the potency of these theories in allaying our anxieties that makes us cling to them so frantically, and that makes our discussions about them so often sterile, and sometimes acrimonious? A number of colleagues have said to me recently: 'But don't you *want* to know what the husband is like?' — and I've found myself saying 'I don't think I do, because that will make it even more complicated'.

One of the things that has struck me since starting back in general practice is the comparatively limited contact we have with our patients in a clinic setting, in terms of both time and scope of knowledge about the patient. This is usually helpful because it is an aid to concentration — how often in general practice one is confused by endless other issues such as physical problems, family problems and work problems. It is impossible to have a comprehensive knowledge of another person. It is like a needle stuck in the groove of a record—the marriage, relationship or indeed development of the individual is a continuing process and all we can do as doctors is to give the needle a bit of a shove. We cannot hope to hear the whole record, but we can ask ourselves what is the most efficient way for *this* doctor, trained in *this* way, working in *this* setting with *these* patients to give that shove? Perhaps this will give us the courage to drop our theories and look at what is happening.

I believe that patients can be helped both by treatment as individuals and as couples, but the techniques used are different; when we are with couples our job is to facilitate communication between the individuals, and we do this at a different level from that at which we work with individuals.

I have looked at the last 100 cases I have seen and I find they confirm two aspects of my work that I suspected: (1) My Balint training has had a profound effect and I do still believe that it is often best to treat the patient who presents. (2) I have difficulties with the joint interview.

Of my last 100 cases, 68 presented with the woman walking into the room alone. Of these 68 the husband was subsequently seen on only seven occasions. Does this mean that the presentation of these patients to this doctor in this setting was the most efficient for treatment? Or that the doctor depended too much on the theory that one should treat the patient who presents? To try to throw some light on this I looked at the reasons why husbands *were* seen.

Husbands of females presenting alone

1. Husband came for vasectomy counselling.
2. Husband in car.
3. Wife said he wanted to come.
4. Wife brought him and said I wanted to see him!
5. Wife asked if I could see him.
6. Husband 'pushing to come in' (waiting downstairs).

As this list shows my notes revealed only the most superficial reasons. What did it mean to these men to be included in the treatment, and what did it mean to the others to be excluded? How many of the others wanted or needed or should have been offered treatment? I am sure most of you can think of cases of non-consummation where the husband got worse as the wife appeared to get better. I can remember very vividly a case I had when I first started this work.

Case Studies

Mrs P.

Mrs P. complaining of non-consummation, had already had her hymen stretched under anaesthetic when I saw her. I worked with her for some time, exploring her vivid fantasies of a tube extending for ever inside, and the fear of her organs, especially her liver, being damaged. Self-examination was easy and revealing and she and I were confident she would succeed. However, her husband developed back trouble and lost all interest. I left the district and the last I heard was that she had had another stretch. There was, needless to say, nothing to stretch, as she admitted three fingers with the greatest of ease.

Mrs W.

The dilemma of when to send for the absent partner is also shown in this patient. Mrs W. came to a family planning clinic for her pill. She told me of the non-consummation of her recent marriage. She is a small thin-faced, timid-looking girl, whose power quickly became apparent when I found myself driving her home a considerable distance out of my way, and writing myself notes to ensure that I arrived on time for her appointments. She is also always on top when they try to have intercourse! She has intense fantasies about her smallness which self-examination has done little to dispel; recently, she let me know that it is not only she who expects intercourse to be painful, but her husband also expects it to be painful for *him*. Should this be taken as evidence that he needs treatment, and if so, should strenuous efforts be made to see him, or would this be an easy way out of the anxiety generated in the doctor by this patient who believes her hymen to be like a Polo mint?

When couples presented together the situation was different. Twenty of my 100 presented as couples, but only six of these were seen together on each occasion, the others being seen in varying combinations of single and joint interviews.

It appears that my anxieties about the joint interview have largely overridden my belief in the theory of treating those who present. Firstly, with couples one cannot use some of the tehniques that we use with individuals, for instance, in the case of frigidity in the interview. With a woman alone one can try to wait out the coldness, suffering the lack of warmth, waiting for a glimmer of real emotion. With a couple I find the husband cannot allow me to do this. He has to butt in, perhaps to 'help' the doctor, perhaps because he cannot tolerate the atmosphere. The other situation is when it is the doctor who cannot tolerate the atmosphere. I find it particularly difficult if one partner is excessively aggressive, especially if the other appears unable to retaliate.

Case Study

Mr and Mrs B.

Mr and Mrs B. came together on several occasions. As soon as they entered the room together Mrs B. started attacking Mr B., spitting her scathing words with venom. He would sit plethoric and asthmatic in his polo-necked sweater, clearly vexed but saying nothing. I tried to see her alone but he would come bursting back into the room. It was not until I arranged for him to see a colleague that Mrs B. and I both really felt free to get down to work on her many problems. Her complaint was of having 'gone off sex, just like that' four weeks after marriage. She remembered thinking 'I've got my man, I don't have to do it again'. Her mother and her grandmother had very negative attitudes towards sex and Mrs B. still expected adults to be perfect and make the world perfect for her. She had a lot of work to do in taking responsibility for her non-sexuality, but I am glad to say that once Mr B. was offered help with *his* problems she worked well and is now considerably improved.

This leads to another difficulty: complications implicit in the joint interview. It is difficult enough to watch what is happening between the doctor and the patient, much more difficult between three. The sort of thing I am thinking of is mutual projection (Main 1966). I do believe that in many marriages this mechanism of unconscious projection of part of oneself on to the other partner, and then hating it in them, is very evident. However I have only really recognised it in one or two cases where I have seen one partner and my colleague the other, and I am convinced that it is best dealt with by helping the individuals to contain more of those parts of themselves that they dislike and despise. It may not be amenable to explanation in a joint interview.

Finally, I want to say a word about pain. There is no question that couples can often say things in front of a third party that they have not been able to say alone, but what they say is still often tempered by a fear of hurting or being hurt too much, and I don't think it is easy to get at the inner unrecognised pain with the partner present. I believe that the old adage is as true in psychosexual medicine as it is elsewhere. One can cure sometimes, relieve often and comfort always. But one cannot comfort unless one gets somewhere near the real pain (even then there are sometimes things in ourselves which prevent us being able to offer comfort). May I finish by telling you about Mrs F.

80

Case Study

Mrs F.

The patient was a secretary in her early forties. She had pretty grey hair and was attractively dressed, sitting with a tight bright smile and a bit of a giggle. She told me of her many attempts to get help with her frigidity, of her visits to psychologists and psychiatrists both with her husband, by herself and in groups. She had tried a variety of clitoral and intravaginal vibrators. As she came to the end of this recital, she said, with an even brighter smile, 'I wonder, doctor, should I try oral sex?' You can imagine my feeling of hopelessness. However, we sat through a number of sessions, until finally one day she began to talk about the first time she had fallen in love, and the joy of walking hand in hand, and for the first time she was able to cry. There was, of course, no dramatic improvement. She did not suddenly become orgasmic, but there was one small change. She began to be able to deal with her 13-year-old daughter a bit better. There are a number of factors that could have been responsible for this, such as the fact that her son had moved away from home, but it would be nice to think that perhaps the chance to become conscious of, and share with me, her pain and grief over her lost innocence in some way helped her to tolerate her daughter's burgeoning sexuality more equably. I do not think this pain could have been reached in a joint interview.

13

Working as a co-therapist

Katharine Draper

My task is to examine the situation of working with a co-therapist and the behavioural methods of sexual therapy, in the way in which we are trained, that is, the discussion of individual cases.

The work of the Institute has grown from a continuous study of clinical material under the guidance of seminar leaders. In contrast, the work of the behavioural therapists has been founded on theory. In 1966 Masters & Johnson published *Human Sexual Response* which gave a detailed description of the physiological changes that take place in a human being, as a result of sexual stimulation in laboratory conditions. On this theoretical basis a system of treatment of sexual problems was evolved (Masters & Johnson 1970) which was aimed at modifying the sexual behaviour of couples. This treatment was originally carried out in an hotel, removed from the stresses and strains of daily living, work, children and other commitments. It was expensive, and we all know the importance of motivation for treatment. The couples were seen individually for long history-taking and then an agreed programme was drawn up which involved first a ban on intercourse and a return to caressing and stroking of non-genital areas, known as sensate focus, then a gradual progression through genital stimulation and sometimes oral intercourse to full vaginal penetration. A special technique, the 'squeeze', was advocated for premature ejaculation. In the residential course, progression through these stages took place over a matter of days. The directions given to the couples were designed to restructure their sexual behaviour but counselling sessions were also used to improve communication between the couples and the same-sex therapist was meant to be the advocate of an 'oppressed' partner in joint sessions. Under these conditions some successful and much publicised results were achieved.

In this country the scheme of treatment has been modified for use on an out-patient basis — the results of a clinic run on these lines have been described by Bancroft (Bancroft & Coles 1976). I was asked to be a co-therapist in a unit which had six couples of therapists. Two couples were based 'in the community', carrying out one of the intentions of the reorganisation which was to integrate the community and hospital arms of the National Health Service. Several teams have no medical member, and in a teaching hospital there are some frequent changes of staff which include social workers, psychiatric social workers (PSWs), psychologists, medical housemen and registrars. I worked for the first year with a clinical psychologist.

Our clinic was held in a community welfare clinic just off the local high street, an hotel converted by two women philanthropists at the beginning of the century, with 'Welcome' in mosaic just inside the front door; opposite was a yard which had stables for the local 'Steptoes', so we were truly 'in the community'. The clinic was held weekly and before starting all the therapists were given a treatment scheme. At the first session each patient had a long interview with the 'same-sex' therapist, having previously filled in a form with details of work, education, family history and then a description of their complaint, hobbies, and smoking and drinking habits. The therapists had a four-page form to complete elaborating these facts, and also including information about sexual experience and arousal. After the interview the therapists conferred and then the couple were seen together and were given instructions, which were usually that there should be a ban on intercourse, and a sheet describing sensate focusing — the couple being expected to have regular sessions of stroking and caressing, which they took in turns in initiating. They were given a sheet with squares to mark their activity and enjoyment for each day (a score of one-five for grades of pleasure). This was intended to be filled in separately by each partner.

At the return visits the homework sheets were commented on and the patients' difficulties were discussed. A general programme of instruction sheets was followed through genital focusing to intercourse. My co-therapist gave all the instructions and he was very enthusiastic about his therapies. I would intervene to interpret some of the interactions which took place during the interview.

In practice I often felt that it was necessary to see the woman on her own for more than the initial interview and, after complying with the request to complete the forms for one or two patients, I discarded the practice in favour of letting the patients tell me their story in the way that seemed important to them. Time spent in form filling gave one no opportunity to talk to them.

When someone else is conducting the interview it is certainly easier to observe the patients' reactions both to each other and to the therapist. Sometimes I would intervene to draw attention to what was taking place but I found to my cost that anxieties that can be explored with patients by themselves seem like an attack when they are brought out in a joint session. We were asked to take medical students who were attached to the psychiatric unit — and a same-sex student sat in at the single interview with the same-sex therapist. This meant that at the joint session there were two therapists, two students and the couple — which made quite a crowd. After a trial period I declined to have students as I feel that the patients' 'offers' are too delicate to be subjected to the observation of students. But this does of course leave us with the conflict that while we want our students to be aware of psychosexual problems we do not want them as observers in our clinics.

After the first year the clinic was reorganised. My new co-therapist was a PSW and although we followed the scheme of seeing patients individually and then as a couple we were both much more flexible in our approach. We did not use the homework sheets at all as we found that far too many patients regarded this as an intrusion into their privacy and we very seldom used the instruction sheets. We also found it very helpful on occasion to have single interviews with the opposite sex.

Our joint session always had at least one, and sometimes more, women who wanted to be seen on their own because they had not got a partner. On a number of occasions I was asked to examine women when they were being treated by a team which had no medical members, but I only do this now on the condition that if there is something significant in the vaginal examination they will come back; it is not possible to explore all the anxiety or fantasy that may be revealed at one interiew. One such woman was referred to me when she and her husband had repeatedly failed to complete their homework schedules; she was sent along to me for an examination. She was a thin, drab and dreary-looking girl and complained that she never wanted sex and her husband just came home and 'slummocked' in front of the telly. She had conceived at 18; her fiancé then went off and she was terminated as a result of family pressure, although she said she was dragged screaming to the theatre. Afterwards she felt both angry and dirty on being offered an IUD since her only relationship was with the fiancé who had deserted her. Discussion with her therapists had failed to resolve these feelings. She lay on the examination couch quivering and weeping and so I was able to begin to explore her feelings about her vagina and her femininity. After several visits she was able to use tampons and the next visit she came back looking absolutely radiant — she had found the tampon was not wet when she had passed water; she presented, and we discussed, a cloacal fantasy. Further conjoint therapy was unnecessary.

Case Studies

Mr and Mrs W.

We saw this couple during the first year when I was working with a clinical psychologist. They went to see their GP because they said their family life was being destroyed by constant quarrelling, and the GP referred them to the clinic. When they first came to see me they presented very contrasting appearances. He was tall, thin, carefully dressed but always rather trendy. One Sunday I read in the *Observer* that it was all right to wear a suit, provided you wore a polo-necked sweater, and the next week he came wearing a polo-necked sweater! He seemed to be very much an *Observer* Review kind of man. His wife, on the other hand, was a dark, pleasant-faced woman with long untidy hair, overweight and wearing an extraordinary garment that looked like a child's outgrown navy school gaberdine. After brief introductions we separated for our single interviews. She had already filled in her form so I knew she came from a medical family; her father was a GP and her brother a surgeon, they had four children aged seven to 16 and she had a university degree. A student was present at the interview but sat quietly at the side.

Mrs W. started by expressing some resentment against the clinic which she said was a depressing place, and about putting her name on the form which she said was like a dossier. She also complained that her husband argued a lot because of their different attitudes to life, that she was placid and easy-going while he was very organised and obsessional. She said that he was a very good interior designer and had won prizes. He was now in practice for the third time, having failed twice before. They were having a very difficult time due to the recession, and had had to reduce his staff so she had had to act as his secretary. She said that he appeared to be self-confident but actually he was taking tranquillisers. Sex, she said, was his 'great beef'; she was very placid in bed and had refused to have premarital sex and the first year of their married life had been embittered because he kept complaining of 'three wasted years'. He devalued their sexual relationship and felt entitled to sleep around although she was not quite clear as to whether he actually did. She was worried about her weight, which he disliked, and she said she was not going to buy herself any new clothes until she got thinner. What she really wanted to do was to write, having got a degree. She did not feel appreciated doing all the housework — rushing round 'like a hen' to tidy the house and the children's mess, which she tolerated happily, before her husband came home. She told me this story passively, sadly, and wept gently at times.

When I examined her she was quite relaxed and detached but she told me she only had a clitoral orgasm. She also complained about her husband's jealousy of the children. He was not 'one of nature's fathers'.

My co-therapist reported that Mr W. (whose forms showed he was the only son of a butcher) complained that he felt middle-aged, the element of excitement had gone out of their marriage and that his erections were not as hard as previously, though sufficient for penetration; he also said that his wife found clitoral stimulation more exciting and had only once or twice had an orgasm from vaginal penetration. He blamed his wife that they did not have a vigorous sex life before marriage. They were both puritanically brought up and religious. He confirmed her remarks that he got tired and depressed from the stresses and strains of work and that he got very irritated with the children's demands. He masturbated two or three times a week and practised oral sex on her but she did not reciprocate.

When we saw them together my co-therapist gave them sheets on non-genital focusing and exaplained the ban on intercourse and asked them to complete the homework sheets separately.

A week later they came back and he presented his homework sheet, which showed that on only three nights had there been any 'activity' and his sheets was covered with all sorts of asterisks and stars which explained that this was due to attendance at meetings, visits from old friends, children's coughs. Finally, they had just decided they would have a session of doing their genital focusing when the telephone rang. She insisted on answering it, he was cross with her and they had had a fiendish row. She had been so upset that she had not completed the forms and she said she was angry about her husband's perfectionist attitudes and disappointed that they did not fit his ideal conception of family life. They had conflicts with the children who would listen to pop music when he expected them to sit down and listen to Beethoven. It was suggested that they should make an effort to go to bed earlier and that he should try and be less rigid with the children. There was apparently considerable conflict in the house as to whether he should go and say goodnight to them with his wife or whether they should all present themselves in the sitting room on the way to bed.

The third interview was more encouraging — their stroking and cuddling sessions had been more frequent and enjoyable and he had been playing with the children. He asked for further instruction sheets and they were given those on 'genital focusing'.

They did not come back until a month later because he had urgent work and there had been a retreat into work tiredness. She said resentfully that he was likely to sit up in bed at 2 a.m. in the morning and say 'Eureka' when he had suddenly solved some problem. She complained that he had never read anything that she had written, and he gave me a lecture on the superior logicality of men's minds, supplementing this with a description of an argument he had had with a well-known writer neighbour; throughout our meetings he was much given to name-dropping.

She came along next time as he had urgent business. She said that genital focusing was not successful because it revealed their 'hang-ups' and that she was very put off by a feeling of observation. But she talked about her feeling that her husband would never change and about his restrictions in childhood when he had had a delicate mother who had insisted that he kept all his Dinky toys wrapped up in tissue paper. She was afraid their marriage would break up, and she felt inadequate in many fields. We went on to talk about her anxiety about her weight; and about her inability to express her femininity and her need to do some work of her own, which her husband resented. On the other hand she was very resentful at his lack of intuition and she expected him to know and understand her feelings absolutely without any explanation. We talked of her fantasy of total empathy.

Our next session was a month later. This time they both attended and reported that they had had an enjoyable camping holiday alone together, though he had still made excessive demands on her in the form of discussing and walking. They were now having intercourse about three times a week. We had a long and, I felt, very critical discussion which centred on their house. It so happened that the evening before I had been looking again at Dr Tunnadine's book (1970), the chapter about symbolism of the vagina and the house. It emerged from our talk that the prize which he had won and which had set him on the road to success had been for their house which was part of a special development, so he expected to be able at any time to conduct important future clients round this showpiece and he expected his wife and his children to live in it rather like little toys, reading the right magazines, playing the right music. We explored the implications of this and he gradually came to appreciate the strain and lack of recognition of their individuality that this attitude imposed on his family.

We had one more meeting a month later. It was summer now and she was wearing a pretty cotton dress, while he seemed much more relaxed. They were getting on well together and when they did have difficulties they seemed able to discuss them, while his relationship with the children was easier. As he had asked for further instruction sheets at an earlier interview I offered them, but he replied firmly that he felt they could now work things out for themselves. We left it that they would phone for another interview if they wanted one but in fact we have not seen them again.

In this case it seemed to me that the early ban on intercourse and joint discussion were a help in easing the tension between them, but that the vital changes were due to their realisation of both their own and each other's fantasies. I was able to work with her feelings about her femininity when he failed to attend, and perhaps it was her altered attitudes which made it possible to discuss his fantasies at a joint session.

It will be noticed that they went from genital focusing to intercourse on their own, without recourse to the sheets, and it was our common experience that couples either made this progress spontaneously, or failed and dropped out.

Mr and Mrs F.

This couple were referred from a nearby teaching hospital because the registrar was very baffled by this nurse in her third year of training who could not consummate her marriage. There was no vaginismus but he offered to do a 'stretch under anaesthetic' if necessary.

I first saw them on my own as my co-worker was away. They came into the small room together, both tall and thin. He was a PhD student, in an anorak and climbing boots; he was more suitably dressed for Hadrian's Wall than for central London. He had a nervous giggle, glasses, short beard, hair on end and 'jack in a box' movements. She on the other hand was dark, pale, with a 'Modigliani' face and a babyish lisp. They told me they were unable to have intercourse and talked of her inhibited family background, that she had been told nothing about sex and that strong religious views had prohibited premarital sex. They had enjoyed petting but they had had absolutely strict 'no go' areas. He giggled a lot and tried to appear self-confident when he told me of the failure of his parents' marriage and how his mother had in fact used him as a confidante while he was in his teens.

He stayed in the room while I examined her. I always leave it to the couples to make their own decisions as to whether they stay or not. She was a bit apprehensive but there was no vaginismus. Despite her nursing training she had absolutely no knowledge of where her own vagina was, and was encouraged to self-examination, but in his presence I did not feel I could explore her feelings and fantasies, nor did I feel that I wanted to break the cocoon that joined them and so I asked them to come back to a joint session. At the next session my colleague saw the husband while I talked to the wife and worked with her feelings about her vagina. She told me that when he had been trying to explore her vagina they had been having a long discussion about a meeting he had been to about the Old Testament, so they had been determined, whatever else they did, to keep their minds on higher things! The husband talked to my co-therapist and was able to express a lot of his anxieties about meeting girls, his feelings that the penis was dirty and the vagina 'clammy'. By the next visit they were playing music instead of having intellectual discussions while they made love; she was using tampons and asked to be fitted with a cap. They are now able to enjoy intercourse and she is using a cap as a contraceptive. I felt that this satisfactory outcome was more easily achieved with a co-therapist because the fantasies of each partner could be explored separately, but we did not use any instruction sheets.

Conclusions

Working in this way has led me to reach some conclusions about behavioural conjoint therapy. First it is expensive of doctor time — with the quadrille of single and joint interviews and therapist consultations, one new and two follow-ups is a full clinic load.

What about the therapist? When the therapist is convinced that they have an effective treatment the onus for recovery is borne by the patients. If progress is not made it is because the patients have not carried out their tasks and they are chided into trying harder. This will increase the feelings of failure in patients who have not benefited because they will feel that it is their fault that they have not benefited from this 'excellent' treatment.

It is certainly less demanding for the therapist to work in this way. It is comforting to share the anxieties aroused by the patient and it is far less exhausting to tell the patients what to do than to work with their feelings and try to understand the doctor-patient relationship.

But we are really here for the patient's sake, so what about the patient? Well, when the difficulty lies in communication between the patients then seeing a couple together can be helpful. Sometimes when one member has been helped by psychosexual therapy, encouragement is needed to share the improvement with the partner.

In couples where the situation has so deteriorated that attempts to make love are fraught with hostility then the 'ban on intercourse' and 'sensate focus' can be helpful. It resembles the time-honoured 'pax!' of children's games and lets the fighting stop and the thinking start.

The difficulties are that this technique can be used indiscriminately. One patient I saw had been given the sheets on sensate focus, having presented with a complaint that she could not bear to be touched! The basic anxieties can be left unaltered, while the unsuccessful patient is left feeling more of a failure than ever. Some patients resent the intrusion of the therapist with the instruction sheets. And, of course, if a patient has no partner, then there is no therapy.

Findings with Patients

Part IV Owning the problem and establishing intercourse

Many patients suffer such acute anxiety over their sexuality that they are too embarrassed to make a verbal complaint; to be able to offer therapy it is necessary to understand the covert presentations of sexual difficulty as Dr Freedman discusses. Obstacles to expressing the problem and finding help were demonstrated in the film 'Breaking the Ice' (Appendix I, p. 238). Despite the more permissive attitudes of contemporary society there are still many couples who fail to consummate their relationship. Dr Bramley's study was designed to evaluate the work of members of the Institute, not as a study of non-consummation, but her results also show the length of time many patients take to find appropriate therapy.

14
Covert presentation of psychosexual problems

'While I'm here, doctor, I don't suppose it matters, but ...'

Roland Freedman

I see patients with sexual problems in two different settings: those who come to me as the doctor of first contact, and those who are referred by other doctors. Patients in this latter group have already revealed, in general terms, the nature of their disability. The first group has a fundamental difference — it consists of patients whose opportunities for revealing their difficulties depend to an almost alarming extent on me. How receptive, how busy, how tuned in, how tired, how 'sympatico' I am with a particular patient may determine whether or not the real reason for consultation will be revealed, perhaps ever.

On going through the notes of the last few patients with sexual problems who have consulted me in general practice, I was struck by the fact that what turned out to be the presented problem was rarely the most important problem. The offer often seemed to serve as little more than a ticket of admission while the real reason for visiting the doctor appeared to have to remain hidden initially.

Michael Balint (1957) made this observation and wrote about it extensively some 30 years ago. I make no apology for reminding you of it, for several very good reasons. Firstly because there is certainly not one of us who, at some time, although listening to what the patient is saying, for some reason or other does not, will not, or refuses to receive the message. We listen but we hear not. I have already suggested why this may be so in my case and I expect the same factors apply to others. The second reason for my reminding you that the real reason for the patient's attendance may be hidden is because if the message is received and understood that in itself can be wonderfully therapeutic.

The third reason concerns two recurring themes at my psychosexual problems clinic. 'I tried to tell him years ago but he wouldn't listen', or 'He didn't seem to understand', or 'He made me feel dirty', or 'Eventually I just had to pluck up courage and ask to be referred'. In these words, or some similar, the complaint is articulated quite frequently. The other theme is a realisation, oft repeated, that this patient is an extension, several months or many years on, of an exactly similar patient seen in general practice in the early stages of the problem. Now the disability has become a way of life, a profoundly miserable way of life at that, and that much more difficult and time-consuming to rectify. If only the doctor had lifted up a corner of the screen hiding the real complaint, what might he have discovered underneath, what fears, what guilt, what ignorance, what anxiety may have had the chance to escape and be shared? Let me give you some examples:

Nigel came about his headaches due, he said, to sinusitis. In passing he mentioned that, although it was not his problem, his wife wondered if something should be done about her vagina as it seemed to have been stretched by childbirth. His own anxieties about his supposedly inadequate erections were more appropriately ventilated. He had used a spurious complaint to gain admission and then invoked the psychological mechanism of 'projection' to approach the real problem.

Denise came about her ears, which, she said, were blocked. I could find nothing abnormal, not even wax. In the course of consultation it came out that she had another 'block' which was much more important to her but too threatening to reveal initially. She had been married for four years and the marriage had not yet been consummated. A few weeks later following further discussion and physical examination it had been.

Robert consulted about having the sebaceous cyst on his neck removed. As he was leaving he inquired as to whether it would be possible to have his vasectomy reversed. No, they had not yet decided to have further children; he was just wondering. His fears about losing his sexual ability in conjunction with losing his fertility soon came out. Apparently he had rushed (or had been rushed) into a vasectomy when their previous method of contraception was proving unsatisfactory.

I would like to tell you in rather more detail about three other patients, each for a special reason. The first two in a sense could be called iatrogenic problems. Certainly medical management had something to do with causing the problems.

Case Studies

Susan

Susan had come because she had been getting stabbing pains in the left side of her head for a few weeks. I had not met her before and knew nothing of her background. She was a woman in her mid-thirties, and seemed rather angry and aggressive. I was unable to find a cause for the pain.

I enquired about her general health. She had been depressed, she said, but had got over it now. As she was the last patient I took the plunge and remarked on her hostile attitude. She responded that she was having an early menopause like her mother did at 36, and had been told that she would have to accept this and come to terms with it. I pointed out that this could have all sorts of implications, not necessarily all bad, but she seemed very unhappy. We discussed her feelings about it. She had been having investigations for infertility for the last 11 years and had now come to accept that she could never become pregnant. She went on to refer to her mother's early menopause being accompanied by going off sex from then onwards.

How about her? Her aggression had melted somewhat by now and gave way to tears. She was having intercourse very rarely because it was so painful. She could hardly remember the last time, probably three months ago. She had been referred to a gynaecologist who had told her she could find nothing wrong and that the problem was possibly in the mind. Susan said she was puzzled by

92

this as she thought this meant she was 'mental'. The feeling she conveyed to me was that she supposed she should not be able to be sexual, also of such anger about her reproductive lot that she jolly well was not going to be sexual. We talked about these feelings and the assumptions she seemed to be making about her sexual adequacy. Yes, she had been distressed, even enraged by her failure to conceive, but that was over and she had come to terms with it. In any case sex used to be enjoyable and not painful. I believed her but was still left with this attitude of hers that she was not now equipped for sex.

It seemed an appropriate time to perform a gynaecological examination, at the same time discussing with her the impression I had that she seemed to be assuming that she could no longer be a sexual woman. Although she had been examined previously this had been to establish the absence of pathology. Now the examination was being used to reinforce my suggestions about her absence of periods, her absence of fertility and her mother's absence of sexuality having nothing to do with her sexuality. I was endeavouring to convey to her that nothing she had told me, or that I had discovered on examination, in any way pointed to her being other than a complete sexual woman.

I must have been fairly successful in this because she came back a few weeks later saying that their sex life had been transformed. She also expressed her astonishment that she could have changed so dramatically straight after one consultation.

What can be learnt from this? Perhaps that it is worthwhile using one's imagination in an attempt to unearth tacit assumptions and then to ventilate them; that only then is it possible to reassure effectively; that, although it is difficult, if not impossible, to do this within the confines of a ten-minute consultation, it need not take a disproportionate amount of time. And, finally, that although female doctors may often be the best people to deal with female problems, male doctors may sometimes have the edge on them in being better able to convey to a woman that she is sexual or is still sexual.

Jane

The next patient was in her late twenties and had been referred to my outpatient clinic by her G.P. She had consulted her doctor because on her oral contraceptive she had been having irregular bleeding and also kept getting attacks of thrush. The doctor suspected that there was a more distressing problem which was not being presented. She had soon uncovered the patient's sexual unhappiness and dyspareunia and wondered if these were the result of her recurrent thrush.

The patient told me that she had had a very satisfactory sexual relationship during the first four years of her marriage. She had had her second baby three years ago and since then had been off sex. Her recollection of the events at that time were distressing to her. She had, she said, been forced to use a bed-pan and her labour had been a degrading experience. The physical details may not be important — what is important is the feelings she had about these events. Now she could hardly bear her husband to come near her and intercourse was occurring less than once a month, and only as a duty.

Up to then she had loved the notion of having babies and had never had negative feelings about this. Now she had a conviction that if she did become pregnant her body would reject the baby. We explored together her feelings about being damaged and defiled and she of course now readily understood why she was rejecting sex. With the help of a physical examination (the body-mind approach again) the light at the end of the tunnel was beginning to come into sight.

Matthew

Matthew complained of being unable to cope effectively with his work as a solicitor. He said his performance had deteriorated and that it seemed to be getting worse. He gave the impression of being a rather ineffectual character who had become despondent over his lack of success. We discussed his depression and I decided that drug treatment was not called for, but I would see him again. As he was leaving he casually remarked that his sex life, which had never been very active, was becoming less so. He had only been married for about six months and his wife was not very happy.

I was not at all surprised about his sexual inadequacy although I had completely failed to pick it up. It seemed in keeping. I started 'treatment' by studying the problem with him and saw him on two subsequent occasions. On the second of these the results of tests which I carry out routinely in all cases of impotence were back. His serum prolactin was enormous, several hundred thousand.

He had also developed what he described as weakness of his right eye. Clinical examination revealed a right temporal hemianopia and incoordination of his right hand. His pituitary tumour was subsequently removed.

Perhaps the lesson to be learnt here is that however characteristic of psychosexual abnormality a case of impotence may be the possibility of an organic lesion must be excluded. Extremely uncommon they may be but they will be missed if we omit routine screening. Although our training is firmly, and rightly, based on an understanding of the doctor-patient relationship, we must not forget physical factors. Generally speaking physical factors are more common causes of sexual problems in men than in women, but they are still very rare. What occurs frequently and repeatedly are emotional disorders requiring a sensitive doctor who is able to pick up first signals and who is prepared to tune in to them.

15

Non-consummation

'We've never managed intercourse'

H. Morag Bramley

We all love a wedding. This is one of the happiest occasions in our society. The rejoicing, the congratulations, speeches wishing them a happy future and the eventual send-off, give the couple that happy thrill that at long last they will be really together. What a heartbreak and a disaster if the honeymoon is a disappointment and a misery. With what disappointment and sense of failure do the couple return to start their new life, a big cloud between them which they hope no one will see. They've never managed to have sexual intercourse.

Case Studies

A woman who had to have an emergency admission to hospital

One such couple, Mr and Mrs Sprite, both civil servants and aged 27 years, suffered their misery for three years until one night the emergency doctor used by her GP was called at 2 a.m. Mrs Sprite, who was on an oral contraceptive, complained of lower abdominal pain and bleeding on the fourteenth day of her cycle. Without vaginal examination by the emergency doctor she was admitted to a gynaecological ward. The house doctor was unable to do a vaginal examination and she was discharged the next day as the bleeding and pain had stopped. She was given a gynaecological out-patient appointment where a young doctor tried to examine her without success. She was sent to my clinic with a history of pelvic pain, intermenstrual bleeding and non-cooperation in vaginal examination. Had the emergency night admission been a cry for help since she had been too shy and frightened to mention her inability to have sexual intercourse to her GP when she had gone for her pills?

She presented as a tall, elegant, well-groomed girl who, when she began to relax and was encouraged to talk freely, told me that her mother had been embarrassed trying to talk about periods and that she herself had been too embarrassed to tell anyone that she'd never had intercourse in three years of marriage. Sex in marriage, according to her mother, was for having babies and not for pleasure or love, and there had been grave warnings about not getting into trouble before marriage.

She started to sweat when I suggested that she get on to the couch and when on it she said she felt sick and I got her a drink of water. She said she'd always had pain when penetration had been attempted and she gave me a strong feeling that there was something terrible about her genital area, which was indeed a reflection of what she felt about it. With a bit of coaxing she moved herself down the couch on to the finger I'd laid on her vulva. With my finger in her vagina I suggested to her that her feelings of faintness, sickness, pain, etc., were her feelings about the rightness and legitimacy of sexual enjoyment when no pregnancy was being desired or sought. There was silence.

I invited her to feel inside herself which she did very tentatively — she told me that it was slippery and all right and she then looked very pleased with herself. She had never dared to touch that area before or attempted to insert a tampon. Later she told me that all the way home she'd been saying to herself in a delighted way: 'I've done it, I've done it — I've put my finger inside'.

She returned in a month to discuss with me how she'd enjoyed sex and even visited her GP to have a cervical smear without difficulty. She was sure it was her mother's inhibitory attitude that had been holding her back.

Mrs Sprite's need for another kind of mother was made clear to me when I found myself running for a drink of water, thinking of her as a girl rather than a woman and encouraging her to touch her vulva and vagina. She was able to use this relationship to free herself from her own mother's inhibiting precepts and to take a step further into adulthood. To be allowed or rather encouraged to examine herself had also contributed to her acceptance of her body and her desires as good.

How long would it have taken her to go to her GP and ask for help if she'd not presented by this dramatic method of emergency night admission to hospital?

A woman who had to keep people at arm's length

Mrs Brown, a 38-year-old, well-dressed, professional woman, married for 15 years, complained that she had never been able to have proper sexual intercourse. She had a happy family of four adopted children. She sat down beside me in a businesslike way and took charge of the interview, talking rapidly so that I could hardly say a word. The interview was almost over when I realised that no vaginal examination had been done. On examination she had extreme vaginismus.

I asked the patient why she had to control her husband and keep him out as she was now controlling me and keeping me out of her vagina and out of the conversation. She said she was afraid of pain because she was abnormal and something was wrong down below. Then followed a long story of visits to hospitals, infertility investigations and then the adoption of children. Recently she had been sent to a gynaecologist because she had a thrush infection and her GP had said she was abnormally tight. At the visit to the gynaecologist she was anaesthetised, stretched, and woke with a dilator in her vagina which she found very distressing. This confirmed in her mind that there was something very abnormal about her.

When I told her the reality — that she was using normal vaginal muscles to keep her husband and me out and that physically she was quite normal — and when she examined herself with her fingers, she was really amazed. She went away and practised stretching herself and came to terms with the fact that her genitals were normal.

Other factors in her childhood had also made her feel abnormal. She was illegitimate and had spent time and effort as a schoolgirl trying to hide this fact with fears that anyone who came too near would find out that she was different. This and the abnormal vagina had fused in her mind. She had a fantasy that abnormality in her background and physical abnormality in her genitals had made intercourse impossible.

In my relationship with her, she was keeping me at arm's length — and her dawning awareness of this enabled her to talk about her need to keep others, including her husband, from getting too near her lest they should find out the abnormal things about her. Facing her with self vaginal examination was crucial to her coming to terms with reality, and her feelings of something wrong below were in fact a reflection of her feelings about herself as an illegitimate child.

After three sessions of one hour each, she described how at last they were having full intercourse with pleasure after 15 years of non-consummation, which she could hardly believe.

The second marriage of an older man

Mr Rook, a healthy, fair, stocky 58-year-old man, said he'd seen an article in the newspaper about the psychosexual clinic and had come for help. He had complained to his GP about his lack of potency and had been given Potensan Forte on two occasions, but he was still unable to have intercourse with his new wife whom he'd married after four years as a widower. He looked very uncomfortable and shy; he'd never discussed such a thing with a woman — he'd never even talked about sex with his first wife although they'd had regular intercourse for 26 years.

He refused examination and this made me aware that he was relating to me as a woman or mother figure rather than as a medical doctor. Gradually he relaxed and expressed his feelings of ignorance beside his wife who wanted sex in novel and exciting ways which he did not think were proper. He felt he could not discuss these things with her and, in the same way, he was obviously having difficulty in discussing them with me.

It seemed odd that a man who had had regular sex for 26 years could be ignorant, but it became apparent that this was defence against his anxieties about his inability to satisfy his new wife. He also had anxieties about his daughter of 15 years, who might disturb them while they were having intercourse. He was dubious about the propriety of exciting sex at his age, while his first wife was in her grave and of the offence he might cause his teenage daughter.

This man made me feel like a mother or authority figure (although I was younger than him). In this context he was able to free himself from his negative feelings about his sexuality, his age and the fact that he was a widower. I also suggested that some discussion with his daughter about her feelings might be helpful.

He thanked me effusively as he left and I felt that here was a man who wanted to please women. He wanted very much to please his sexually adventurous wife and yet felt terrible anxiety about displeasing his daughter by being improper at his age. These anxieties perhaps had produced his impotence. Two visits later, he reported that he was able to have intercourse, and rather shyly said his wife was teaching him many new things and he was very happy. He seemed also to have resolved his problems with his daughter.

A couple who hoped for 13 years that it might happen

Gladys at 23 years old had helped her mother bring up seven younger children. She was a good little 'mother' but had been given no information about sex. She looked forward to having her own children but after marriage to Mr Jones and all its exciting hopes, bitter disappointment resulted for her and her husband. The first attempt at sex had been very painful and so she had tightened and continued to do so. Her GP gave her tranquillisers but nothing changed. Her husband consulted his GP who said he'd have to go and get help somewhere. They resorted to mutual masturbation. They were so keen to have a family that an adoption society was approached — they refused to help but suggested artificial insemination. They were too shy to proceed with this. After 13 years of this unhappiness, Mr Jones, who was an only child, discovered that his cousin's baby was being taught to call his (Mr Jones's) parents Granny and Grandpa. This triggered some anger and despair in him and, having asked around, he made an appointment himself at a psychosexual clinic. The moment at which a patient presents is often a psychologically vital time for him.

They looked a bedraggled pair when I saw them — she had a dowdy threadbare brown coat and stringy hair, and he a rather scruffy off-white anorak and untidy fuzzy hair. He was a Coal Board fitter of 34 and she a shop assistant of 36. They were very nervous and said it was a great effort to come but they'd never done anything in 13 years and they wanted children.

As I asked her to get on the couch, she said very firmly that the doctor had been unable to do a cervical smear for her. She made me feel that she was very afraid of examination and indeed she had extreme vaginismus. As I laid a finger on her vulva and asked how it felt she described the bleeding, ripping and pain which would have to take place when she first had intercourse and said she was very much afraid of pain. She said she thought she must be abnormal down below, and then added 'I must be abnormal in the head as well to have gone this long'.

After a discussion of her feelings of abnormality both physically and mentally she ventured to put one finger in her vagina and said she would practise doing this.

On the following two visits she looked quite different with a bright orange jumper and neatly done hair. She'd really stretched herself and a vaginal examination was fairly easily carried out. She said she felt enormously better about herself as a woman — somehow she'd grown up. The husband said he'd got partially inside, but was afraid of pushing too hard, hurting his wife and starting all the trouble over again. She said she wished he'd push in spite of her protests. When they left, he said in a much more positive voice, 'We hoped before that some day things would come right, but we had no foundation for this. Now we are hoping with knowledge — we know it will soon come right'.

This woman had made use of the doctor-patient relationship to do the last bit of sexual growing up which lack of parental permission, and fear of pain had prevented her from completing. At the final visit both were smartly dressed and smiling happily. He said they had had enjoyable intercourse every night for the last seven nights and were hoping for an early pregnancy.

Life is not full of successes — it's often a mass of failures. One woman after 30 years' non-consummation came to me determined to achieve intercourse because her husband was paying respects to the priest's housekeeper — who was an ill-organised, incompetent and slovenly woman. I was so blind in the doctor-patient relationship to her manipulating of me and of her husband that, although she finally managed to have sexual intercourse with her husband, I should not have been surprised that the husband did finally go off with the incompetent, non-bossy but warm, loving housekeeper leaving a furious, 'after all I've done for you', competent wife behind.

Assessment

A group of Institute members decided to try and assess the results achieved using our seminar training methods. Non-consummation was chosen as a condition for study. A pilot project published by Bramley et al. (1981) was reproduced in full in Freedman (1983).

We mounted a further Nuffield-supported prospective study on non-consummation which is not yet published and in which we used an outside assessor of our results instead of controls — the difficulties of using controls being explained in the pilot study. The assessor corroborated our findings — visiting individual couples before and after treatment.

Some of the results are as follows: 159 couples were prospectively entered by 16 seminar-trained doctors instructed for three separate days in the research method to be used in their own clinics over 27 months (1978–80).

The cumulative consummation rate was 72 per cent at 24 months. Male impotence was a contributory factor in non-consummation in 30 couples — sometimes a primary cause and sometimes secondary to vaginismus. These couples did not do worse than others. The average duration of symptoms was four years' non-consummation but the length of symptoms did not seem to affect the result.

Twelve couples were first presentations and 253 agents including 54 NHS consultants had been visited by the other 135 couples. The number of agents consulted did not seem to affect the consummation rate which was highest in those consulting three or more agencies. An average of three hours was spent by the doctor on the 95 couples consummating in six months and three and a half hours for those who did not.

It was not necessary to insist on the partner's presence in this treatment and those women who presented and attended on their own had a better result at six months than the others. Eight women conceived ten times without penetration and their consummation rate was poor. Fantasies often play a large part in the course of vaginismus and non-consummation. Many were expressed by patients including fears of smallness, damage, etc. Twenty-three women complained of traumatic experiences which contributed to their consummation difficulties and which they had attributed to medical encounters.

In spite of doing this Nuffield study, no questionnaires for the patients were used lest they interfere with the delicate doctor-patient relationship. We collected data, but uppermost was our main concern — the use of a good doctor-patient relationship for:

1. Understanding the cause of the patient's difficulties, for example in Mrs Brown who kept me out of her conversation and her vagina and thus helped me to realise her need to keep people away from her.
2. Helping sexual maturing and growth, as with Mrs Sprite who could only make her 'terrible' needs known by emergency admission to hospital. She had to grow and accept her own adulthood and decisions and leave parental injunctions behind.

Part V Women patients

Frigid Wives
Although working with each patient is a unique presentation, it has been observed that patterns of sexual difficulty emerge. The papers in this section report studies that have been made of certain groups of patients, some classified by the presenting symptom and others by the maturational stage at the time of the complaint. These have been amplified by relevant case studies, of varying lengths, taken from other papers. The topics that are covered are those that have stimulated individual doctors to review and report their work; I have attempted to arrange them in a logical sequence, but they do not aim to give a comprehensive account of sexual difficulties. The early work of members of the FPA was all with women patients, so that their studies of non-consummation, frigidity and 'contraception and sexual life', described in the Introduction, had been published before the clinical meetings reported here; these papers therefore represent only a partial account of their work with women. The first paper in this section is a reassessment of their previous analysis of frigidity by Dr Blair and Dr Pasmore.

Sexual Difficulty after Childbirth
I have placed these papers as a separate group because this is not only the most frequent cause of secondary frigidity but it is also a time when the patient is in regular contact with doctors, whose interventions at this critical maturational time can affect her subsequent ability to be a mother and a wife. Two papers are followed by a brief case study, given 'off the cuff' at a meeting, which I have included because it is typical of numerous clinical encounters.

Psychosomatic Pelvic Pain
The laparoscope has shown that many women, previously diagnosed as suffering from 'pelvic congestion' have normal pelvic organs but the enigmatic pain remains though the organs are seen to be healthy. The extract, from a paper by Dr Tobert, serves as an introduction to this subject, and is followed by a paper by Dr Blair and case studies.

Hysterectomy
The recent growth of post-hysterectomy self-help groups is evidence of the confusion, anger and sorrow that many women feel after this operation. On the other hand some women will meno-'rage', with physical complains (and menorrhagia), to achieve the termination of unwanted feminine functions. These emotional concommitants of hysterectomy are studied in two papers and a 'cautionary' case study.

16

Frigid wives: a revised classification

Margaret Blair and Jean Pasmore

Frigidity includes all degrees of disinclination or lack of sexual response in a woman, from failure to achieve mutual orgasm during intercourse to the total rejection of any sexual approach. It is taken to imply an emotional response, and cases where it is a temporary disturbance due to external events, e.g. physical illness, bereavement, anxiety due to economic crises, etc., are not considered in this paper.

In 1964 we wrote a paper summarising the work of eight family planning clinic doctors, who had met weekly for five years under the leadership of the late Dr Michael Balint, to discuss cases of frigid women (Blair & Pasmore 1964). About 80 per cent were easily fitted into the clinical classification proposed.

Four main groups and some sub-groups were defined showing a graduation from Category 1 the least ill, to Category 4, the most difficult to reach.

Summary of the four original categories
Category 1
Newly married couples having difficulties in the transition to married life.
Category 2
Women *uncertain* of their femininity.
Category 3
Women who are *angry* about their femininity.
Category 4
Patients with overwhelming sexual anxieties who deny all feelings.

Detailed explanation of the 1964 categories
This is necessary before we consider the reasons for using instead a modified classification which better reflects underlying problems rather than symptoms.

Category 1 (eight patients)
All these patients were confident that help would be available and responded quickly to short treatment. The doctor acknowledged the significance of their fantasies about intercourse and their own bodies, and during vaginal examination helped them to accept the reality.

102

These patients showed early and reversible difficulties which, if untreated, might later have placed them in one of the following categories.

Category 2 (26 patients)
These were all uncertain of their femininity, but were sub-categorised according to the way they expressed this uncertainty. They had unhappy childhoods and shadowy husbands, whom we did not hear much about, but a good relationship with children.

Sub-category 2a. These patients complained of *limited* enjoyment in intercourse. These were rather intense and had good relationships with their young babies. Although the husbands were successful, they were seen by their wives as weak. Their fathers had been remote — physically or emotionally — and they disliked their mothers. They described intercourse in terms of something missing — one patient said it was like stretching for an apple, just out of reach. Their capacity for only limited enjoyment was also shown in their relationship to the doctor — they liked coming but remained unchanged. They were easy with their own bodies — making no difficulty in examination and accepting the cap as a method of contraception. Many showed a rich fantasy life which seemed to represent unobtainable relationships which they were unable to renounce in favour of reality.

Sub-category 2b. These patients were able to enjoy intercourse occasionally or only *under certain conditions.* They were boyish, bright and showed feeling. They described stormy childhoods in which father had been an important figure whereas mother was shadowy or disapproving. Their husbands were insignificant figures. Their relationship to their children varied. Some knew under what conditions they could enjoy intercourse but others did not. This group were sometimes able to make use of their fantasies to obtain enjoyment.

Sub-category 2c. These patients showed their uneasiness about their femininity by difficulty with their female bodily functions, e.g. dyspareunia, dysmenorrhoea, recurrent miscarriages, and Caesarean or forceps deliveries. Their childhoods were lonely or strict. Their relationships past and present showed a marked absence of warmth or interaction and they did not make good relationships with the doctor.

Sub-category 2d. These patients showed their uncertainty by their difficulty with the social feminine role. They often could not cook or sew and had little interest in their homes, preferring the masculine world of business or profession. They married late and none of them had children.

Category 3 (16 patients)
These were angry about their femininity. Their childhoods were eventful or traumatic; their husbands resented but respected.

Sub-category 3a. These patients were aggressive. They talked easily and with expression. Although their complaint was of no feeling in intercourse, most had *some* feeling at some time. Four (out of seven) were pregnant before marriage but many of the group did not have a good relationship with their children. Four hated their mothers. They had a significant relationship with their fathers and husbands. They were aggresive towards the doctor. Although some thought their bodies ugly, they gave little detailed information about their fantasies. They were less concerned with their internal world than with their anger at the external world.

Sub-category 3b. These patients showed their anger about being women by being resentful victims. All had been married more than five years when first attending. They had early marriage difficulties and four (out of seven) had never enjoyed intercourse, and blamed their husbands. Their childhoods were unhappy and several had parents who were absent through death or remarriage. They had troublesome children, and were difficult patients who tried to control the doctor. Three described vivid fantasies. They made men helpless and then blamed them for it.

Sub-category 3c (only two patients). These women were using a definite mechanism to express their anger — by confusing. Naturally they did this with the doctor also, so that there was no clear-cut picture to describe. When this defence was interpreted, they began to show characteristics of the other groups.

Category 4 (7 patients)
The anxieties of these patients about their sexual functions were so overwhelming that they denied all feelings. They often showed one of the characteristics of Categories 2 and 3:

They married men older than themselves. They were careful of their appearance, and superficial and inhibited with the doctor, making it difficult to establish contact. There were many physical complaints, especially of difficulty with their genitals. They hid their real anxieties which were denied. These patients give an overall picture of not being able to risk close involvement with any other human being, protecting themselves by withdrawal.

A new classification
In the years since this work was done, there have been two kinds of important change:

Social change
In the intervening 12 years premarital intercourse has become the norm rather than the exception, so that the concept of marriage is regarded as separate from the physical expression. When the paper was written the marriage ceremony symbolised permission for intercourse to take place, but now it is an expression of commitment.

The personal viewpoint of the authors
We have worked in varied settings, and many of our patients have presented with needs other than contraception. Dr Blair works in Charing Cross Hospital, and sees many patients referred for psychosexual difficulties; she has a special interest in requests for termination of pregnancy. Dr Pasmore works at the Cassel Hospital marital clinic, where patients are referred for marital difficulties of all kinds, although many present with psychosexual difficulties as their main complaint. We find that we have both independently arrived at a classification of patients whose main complaint is frigidity, which, in spite of the difference of the settings in which we work, correspond surprisingly closely. We now think in terms of three groups of patients who have problems related to: (a) their ideas about their own anatomy and their ideas about the function of their genitals; (b) difficulty with the social feminine role; and (c)

difficulty in their relationship with men, using the marital interaction as a vehicle for malign projection systems.

Comparing the new classification with the old

We both use this framework in our daily work. It does not contradict the original classification, but rather allows for a less rigid system which, as we said in the original paper, is valuable only as giving a 'clear picture of the predominant situation in the patient's inner and outer worlds as regards her frigidity' at a given moment. Indeed, we have both come to feel that basically frigidity is always an expression of the woman's uncertainty and anxiety about her own femininity, and that the special groups in the original classification represent only the ways in which she defends herself from this anxiety. These ways of expression are constantly changing, especially in therapy, as the underlying anxieties are more nearly approached, and this explains the statement made in the original paper that patients can change from one group to another during therapy.

We can now consider our present standpoint towards each of the categories in the 'old' classification.

Category 1

The social change has a special bearing here. Premarital intercourse is now the rule rather than the exception. It has resulted in far fewer patients presenting with physical difficulties about consummation, although these do still occur. On the other hand, perhaps more confusion occurs about the meaning of marriage and the deeper implications and commitments and dependence involved.

Case Study

Mr and Mrs A. (seen by Dr Blair)

Mrs A. ws referred from an ordinary family planning clinic which she had been attending for four years for the pill. Her complaint was that intercourse very rarely took place and there had been no attempt for six months.

She came to the psychosexual session bringing her husband in with her. He was very defensive at first, saying that he always found it very embarrassing to talk about sexual problems and thought it would be easier to talk to a man. I was able to establish fairly quickly that he had become impotent and this is what he did not like to talk about. He had a number of half-expressed fantasies about 'something being wrong with him'. The couple met when she was 16 and he 17 and both had enjoyed intercourse at first. It had somehow been assumed by both of them and each set of parents that they would progress to engagement and marriage, and Mrs A. presented a rosy and superficial picture of the marriage in which she thought everything except sex was right.

Mr A. was becoming more uncomfortable listening to this, and when I said that I did not think he agreed with her, he started to tell me that their honeymoon was a disaster and sex had never been right since. From that we quickly got on to the meaning, to him, of the marriage ceremony, and it became clear that he had not wanted to get married and felt trapped; but he had to live up to the expectations of his wife and the parents and had gone through the ceremony.

Mrs A. had never realised that he felt like that and was upset and felt rejected, and we talked for a long time about the fantasies of both of them: his about what life might have been like if he had been free — to be irresponsible, leave his job, travel about and meet other girls; and hers about the ideal marriage.

There is a lot of work to be done with this couple, but they left with a better understanding of their problems in relation to reality, and I shall be seeing them again. But this case illustrates very well the difference that 12 years have made, both by social change and to our way of working.

Twelve years ago this couple would probably not have had enjoyable premarital intercourse and would have presented as non-consummation. They would then have been treated, at least primarily, by use of the psychosomatic vaginal examination, which might not have been successful as the problems were not concerned with the wife's fantasies about her own body.

Category 2

The categories still express the predominant situation in a patient's sexual life at the moment of reporting, but we are doubtful about the distinction between sub-categories — 2a limited and 2b conditional. Sub-group 2c however does seem to describe a group of women who have difficulty with their bodily feminine functions and convert their anxieties into actual physical symptoms and signs. This process seems particularly resistant to interpretative psychotherapy, and if one symptom is relieved it is frequently immediately replaced by another physical manifestation. These patients seem to derive considerable vicarious satisfaction from their symptoms and like to talk about them.

Category 2d (social role). The changes in the social climate and the publicity given to Women's Liberation movements have perhaps increased the number of patients who present their difficulties about the social feminine role, and reflect society's confusion over this. In therapy, their attitudes often turn out to be based on their experience of women who have been important to them in their lives — mother, sister, aunt, teacher, etc., and their conflict about these relationships has been intellectually rationalised in terms of the prevailing social ethos. When their conflicts can be shown to be related to these earlier experiences, their present difficulties about their role often fade, and as adults they find themselves able to cope with them.

Category 3

We have both come to the conclusion that anger always covers a patient's feeling of inadequacy as a woman. Perhaps with longer experience we have become more skilled in reaching this uncertainty earlier in treatment, usually in the first interview. As the patients recognise their underlying uncertainties, they find themselves better able to deal with their anger and are not so troubled by it. A minority, however, cannot make this step in understanding their own feelings. They are unwilling to give up the anger which gives them a sense of justification, and they will opt out of treatment rather than accept the underlying feelings.

Case Study

Mrs B. (seen by Dr Pasmore)

Mrs B. was an impressive figure, a Valkyrie, very tall and blonde and completely dominating, who threw at me the problem that she loves her husband very much but can't let *him* make love to her, although she enjoys sex with her lover. She has thought and thought it all out, doesn't understand it, and if she can't find the answer will have to leave him. Her challenging attitude left me no room for intervention, but as she talked she herself became aware of the superficiality of her intellectualisations about her situation. When she told me about her rebelliousness against her mother, who always told her what to do, we saw that her revolt against her husband, against me, and against her mother covered her doubt about her own identity as a woman, and her fear of having her individuality swamped, or of being hurt if she allowed herself to be completely emotionally dependent on anyone. She reacted to this fear by having to be in control and seeing herself as omnipotent, but felt extremely guilty about her destructive use of this power which corresponded to her expectation of being made the victim by anyone else who had power over her. When it was pointed out to her that I had the power to tell her to leave my room at any moment (making it clear that I wanted her to stay), she herself saw the possibility of looking at this power problem in a different way. The fear of dependency became the focus for treatment. At the next session she spoke about her lonely childhood and her feeling that her parents neither understood nor helped her. Her father mocked her for her undeveloped figure. Gradually this needing, weak, fearful, vulnerable part of herself came out, and we saw in a later session how her contempt for this part of herself was matched by her doubts about her unambitious husband. After this, she was able to tell me of an illegitimate pregnancy she had had at 19 and the back-street abortion which she had organised, and the death of the boy involved within a year in a car accident.

On the original classification she presented first of all in terms of symptoms as 2b, conditional, quickly moving to 3a, attacking self or partner. After discussion of the fears which underlay this aggressive attitude, her problems seemed to settle into Category 2d, social role. In our present classification, we would see her main problems as concerned with the relationships of men and women and her fears about dependency (mainly sub-category 2c).

Category 4 (changing feelings)

We are both doubtful about the validity of this category and would see it rather as the extreme of the others. This confirms our original idea that 'during treatment these patients often move into Category 2 or 3'. It may be that we are now more able to find and get in touch with the 'points where feelings are shown'.

Conclusion

Whereas the old classification is in terms of the patient's presenting symptom, the newer one, we hope, more nearly reflects the underlying problems which give rise to these same symptoms.

107

17

Sexual difficulty after childbirth

(i)

Postnatal loss of libido

Alexandra Tobert

Failure to regain sexual happiness after the birth of a baby is a complaint which causes great distress and may pose a threat to the stability of a marriage and a family. These is no evidence that it has a physiological basis and reassurance that all will soon be well has little foundation in fact. It is generally wise to accept that, if a woman complains, she is in need of help.

In many cases enquiry suggests that loss of libido exists as a remnant of an earlier postnatal depression or as the concomitant of one which has settled into an ongoing chronic state. Sexual unhappiness may, in these cases, be the symptom which is presented when a woman has failed to return to a state of well-being months or even years post-partum and is ashamed to continue to complain of tiredness and tearfulness. A story emerges of a miserable, unapproachable woman trying hard not be perpetually bad-tempered and a puzzled, rejected husband, together unable to offer their child the emotional sustenance on which its future well-being depends.

The treatment of the frigidity overlaps and may be found to have coincided with the treatment of the condition as a whole.

The life histories of these women have, of course, all the diversity of human experience, but there are some persistent patterns which may occur singly or in combination. The need to search for understanding of the individual remains always paramount. Only upon this basic assumption may some areas which require exploration be suggested.

The patient's feelings about herself as a woman
There are some unhappy women for whom the physical and emotional functions of femininity are, in varying degrees, burdensome from menarche to menopause. Painful menstruation, symptomful pregnancy, difficult births, problems of child rearing, form a sad progression towards a suffering middle age. Times of physiological transition become crises of emotional instability. Premenstrual tension, postnatal depression, menopausal misery occur singly or coalesce into a pattern. Frigidity in all its many manifestations, temporarily or persistently, may

take its place in the symptom complex of troubled femininity. In terms which do not explore, but at the same time do not deny or contradict the analytical understanding of early childhood development, femininity may be likened to an heirloom which requires to be handed on from mother to daughter in an unconscious, intangible ceremonial. Many patients describe how mother died or departed, or lived unloving or unloved or unfaithful, or how she refused to come to her daughter's wedding or to help with the baby. Thus, there is an interruption of the psychological ceremonial and a break in the continuity. In differing ways and for differing reasons the heirloom of femininity was not offered or not acceptable and the daughter is left bereft and unable to function in wholeness. One deeply troubled woman had been describing her demanding, unsupporting mother. When asked about her grandmother she said, despairingly, 'Like my mother, only more so'.

The patient's feelings about herself as a mother

The demands made upon a woman by a new baby necessarily draw upon her emotional reserves. Hopefully, these reserves have been laid down in childhood, restocked from fulfilling relationships throughout life, and consistently replenished in marriage by a loving husband whose affection she is able to accept and absorb.

It is one of the tragedies of postnatal loss of libido that a woman finds herself compelled to reject sexual love and tenderness at a time when she needs it most. There are among this group of patients many women who have not themselves passed through an experience of mothering which they are then able to re-enact for their children. They are thus faced with the emotional parallel of trying to feed a baby from an empty breast.

Case Study

Heather is 26, plump and pretty. She has been married for seven years and has two daughters aged four years and 18 months. She came because since the birth of her second child, she has lost all interest in sex, feels miserable and realises that her marriage, which had before been warm and happy, both sexually and generally, is deteriorating. She is also worried because she finds herself readily loving to the baby but short-tempered with her older child.

We talked. Gradually understanding began to grow. During her second pregnancy her parents had separated. Logically she thought that this was a good thing because they had fought all their lives, but to her surprise she found herself very upset and her parents constantly on her mind both in the present and in memories of her childhood. She described her father as a drinker and a liar and her mother as a nagger. Many incidents emerged of her mother's coldness and lack of sensitivity to the feelings of her family. Neither parent offered physical affection. Heather is the oldest of three girls. Much had been expected of her regarding sensible adult behaviour. She felt very responsible for her sisters. She depicted with modest pride the contrast both materially and emotionally between her squalid childhood home and the home which she and her husband have created, and she is terrified now of spoiling it by her coldness to her husband and her irritability with her older daughter. She was particularly shocked when she heard herself saying to her husband 'Get off, it's my body, not yours' in the same tone which she had heard her mother use, when as a child, she had pulled the blankets over her head so as not to hear her parents quarrelling.

She has come to see that her childhood provided a poor foundation for her adult femininity, but that her own quality of personality had been sound enough to overcome these handicaps until, at the vulnerable time of her second pregnancy, her parents' separation had disturbed the balance. She also believes that she is treating her elder daughter as she felt that she had been treated herself, by denying her the opportunity of being a child.

Sexually and in her everyday life, Heather became happier. The process of rebuilding her confidence took time, but when she was discharged she was an attractive, self-assured woman, facing the future with optimism.

The patient's feelings about herself as a wife

It is a sad feature of our culture that the daily life of a woman running a home and looking after her husband and children is regarded by some — men and women — as a relegation to a backwater of life and outside the swim of things.

For women who have gained status and satisfaction from their working lives the restrictions imposed by a baby can readily lead to jealousy of the freedom apparently enjoyed by the man of the house. This is particularly likely where there has been an earlier competitiveness with men and a consequent sense of having lost the battle. Sexual activity may then lose its quality of joyful sharing between equals and become instead an imposition to be resisted. It is these women who often make use of those expressions of bitterness and resentment which have become part of our language: 'He takes me for granted, he only wants me for sex.' 'I feel used.' 'He has the best out of life — men always do.' 'Sometimes I give in.'

The patient's feelings about the baby as a reminder of other significant babies in her life

There is a group of women for whom their own baby represents, on an unconscious level, a younger sibling who aroused feelings which could not be expressed or resolved. It is almost inevitable that an older child should feel jealousy and anger, often of great intensity, towards a new baby, but it is not easy for parents (particularly those who have not read the psychology books) to love and support a child through such feelings which must then be repressed and covered by 'good' feelings. Sometimes depression results, but commonly there is the development of personality which is self-disciplined, hard-working and orderly and which functions fully and effectively. Vulnerability lies in situations which provoke dependence and guilt.

Against such a background, the arrival of a baby, with the accompanying relaxation of defences, may reawaken the old repressed feelings and result in all or part of a post-partum symptom complex of depression, withdrawal from offers of affection, anger towards the child and intense anxiety. Not only are these symptoms distressing in themselves, but the contrast they provide to the earlier personality lead to the further distress of self-condemnation.

Case Study

Clare was a young teacher who was seen when her first baby Emma was eight months old. She had been clinically depressed almost immediately after Emma's birth and had been treated with antidepressants. She had improved and was now looking after her baby very well, but she remained tense, anxious and tearful and had lost all her previously healthy sexual feelings. Above all, she was deeply distressed by the feelings of resentment and occasionally near violence which she had experienced towards Emma. 'That isn't me', she repeated.

She had taught, with evident effectiveness, until she was seven months pregnant. Emma was a much wanted child. He husband was also a teacher who proved to be unfailingly loving although much absorbed in his own work. She spoke with deep affection of her own mother and of her happy childhood. She had one sister, three years younger, who had been a sickly, crying baby. Clare had few memories of her early childhood but often said that she was thought of as being a very good child.

110

It proved necessary to work slowly to help Clare to accept her own aggressive feelings which had appeared so out of place in her kindly childhood home and too frightening in their intensity to be expressed towards her sister. She has recently had her second baby and says that she cannot believe that she could feel so different and so warm and patient towards a baby.

Bereavement

Pregnancy is a time of particular vulnerability and the impact of events which occur at this time is likely to be of deep and long lasting significance.

Mourning during pregnancy imposes a conflict which is sometimes almost insoluble. No way may be found to accommodate both the appropriate sadness and gladness except by the denial of all feeling. Then depression is likely to follow. There are among the patients who present with secondary and particularly post-partum frigidity, many who have suffered a bereavement.

Case Study

Margaret ws a woman of 30 who presented with total loss of sexual feeling. She thought that this had been present throughout the nine years of her married life, but on further enquiry it emerged that she had been happy in the early months of her marriage but then her mother had died just before she realised that she was pregnant. She had not been able to tell of her pregnancy and had grieved that her mother had not known of a longed-for grandchild.

During treatment she talked little about sex, but much about her childhood and her mother. To her surprise she discovered a reawakening of her sexual feelings.

Childbirth

There are some women for whom the experience of childbirth is accompanied by almost unbearable feelings of physical and emotional exposure as well as loss of dignity and control. Their fear of 'letting go' tends to make them irritable and irritating patients and thus to test the sensitivity of the most kindly nurses and doctors who themselves, together with other efficient and self-reliant women, often share this sort of personality.

In treatment there is sometimes the need to go over the events of the birth, detail by detail. It seems that the experience cannot be left behind until it has been expressed and shared verbally and emotionally in a way that was not possible while it was happening.

Other childhood traumata

Case Studies

Eileen

Eileen was referred when her third child was three months old. She had become severely depressed within a week of his birth, but refused both antidepressant treatment and hospital admission. Her marriage had been warm and happy both sexually and in other respects, but she had now lost all her responsiveness. The relevance of her own early life experience soon became strikingly apparent.

When she was ten months old, and still breastfed, she was found to have an orthopaedic deformity, and was admitted to hospital, where she remained with occasional short returns home until she was almost three. She was immobilised for most of this time in plaster from her axillae to her ankles. After her return home she developed well in a caring family. She was always determined to be self-reliant and kept her feelings largely to herself, and there was no outward effect of the long maternal separation, until her third child was found to have the same orthopaedic defect. Then it seemed that she was overhwelmed by the full impact of her own infant experience. In this case the treatment required was long-term psychotherapy during which she relived in great detail the desperate fear and misery of the many months in hospital. Gradually the depression passed and sexual interest returned but not as yet to its former joyfulness.

Brenda

Brenda had been sexually accepting, but unenthusiastic when she was just married. After the birth of her first child, she could not bear her husband to touch her. Her thoughts turned frequently to her mother for whom she had a great affection. She compared, with feelings of guilt, her mother's unhappy lot to her own potential but unrealised happiness. When a sound doctor-patient relationship had been established, she told of her childhood memories of her father who had been a heavy drinker and had returned from his drinking sprees to assault his wife and make sexual advances to his daughter.

Many feelings had to be explored, but gradually she found a new and fulfilling sexual happiness and began to relate to her mother in friendship, no longer based on guilty self-denial.

Treatment

The foundation and the framework of treatment must rest upon a sound relationship between a woman and her chosen helper. Within this relationship, she will be able to express her feelings and verbalise her thoughts and memories, so that her story will unfold of its own accord. Diagnosis and treatment will proceed at the same time, as therapist and patient gain insight and understanding together. Within this setting it is hoped that the patient will find a renewed sense of her own femininity and her capacity for self-expression and be able to use these to enrich her sexual life. The focus of treatment remains circumscribed and progress is often achieved with surprising rapidity.

Possible preventative measures

Much work remains to be done to discover whether some patients at risk may be identified antenatally and whether appropriate support offered at that time may mitigate against later difficulties. The type of support requires to be the subject of further research, perhaps along the lines suggested by Frommer (Frommer & O'Shea 1973) and is likely to demand the mobilisation of available resources, possibly through the medium of case conferences involving those concerned with antenatal and postnatal care.

Conclusion

Marital disharmony is prevalent and the divorce rate among parents of young children is continuing to rise, bringing in its wake an incalculable sums of human distress. It is difficult to doubt that the experience of a rich and fulfilling sexual life shared by husband and wife is an important defence against discontent.

(ii)

Post-partum sexuality

Katharine Draper

Some women resume sexual activity soon after parturition. They may cause problems for those attempting to advice on contraception but have no difficulty with their sexuality and its enjoyment. Most women regard the postnatal examination as an 'MOT test' — it gives them permission to return to an active sexual life. A majority resume love-making with pleasure, but some have difficulties; they don't feel like it. Others, not lacking in motivation, find it painful. Working in a family planning clinic we meet many such complaints. Some are simple cases of discomfort and hesitancy, which quickly resolve when their anxieties are listened to and a perceptive examination and perhaps self-examination are carried out. Other cases are more extreme and I would like to describe several cases and then go on to draw some conclusions.

Case Studies

Mrs W.

Mrs W. came to the 'special' clinic a month ago. She was referred from a family planning clinic for loss of libido when taking oral contraceptives. She was a woman of 34, dark, sallow, and though not bad looking she had a plain appearance, and wore blue and beige clothes. She complained that since the birth of her second child she was not interested in sex and now felt she could scream when she was touched. She was afraid it was breaking her marriage. Her first child was born after eight years of marriage during which sex had been normal (but she had her 'off' days). She had a 'terrible' delivery, extremely painful and was confused and terrified when she didn't know whether to push. She shouted and screamed and was told off for frightening others. After this birth she found intercourse difficult for a year and then it gradually improved.

She had another child because she did not want an only child, attended classes, learnt to relax and was determined to have the baby 'normally'. When the waters broke at home she went to hospital and after some hours she was offered 'hormones' to accelerate the birth — she resisted these adamantly. 'It's my body, I won't have it', she said, but finally was prevailed upon to have a drip and the pains became continuous and painful. She felt that there had been intrusion on her integrity by the doctors forcing their methods on her and cheated of a normal birth. She had a retained placenta and was 'pushed and poked for ages'. Her husband stayed with her during labour but was not present at the birth, 'not a man's place — undignified — not at your best'.

Now, she complains, she feels 'more of a mum' and just can't stand any sexual approach, and though she makes an extra effort to do small things for her husband, such as making cups of tea, he fails to understand that it is 'nothing personal'.

When examined she lay with her hands behind her head and eyes on the ceiling, rather taut and embarrassed. When I suggested she touch herself she said 'It's asking a lot', jumped off the couch and pushed me away.

I have described Mrs W. at some length because she illustrates so many different facets. Before childbirth, intercourse had been sufficiently enjoyable to cause no problem in the relationship, though it did not sound very exciting. That she did not want her husband present at the birth, and resisted self-examination, suggest inner anxiety and a need to preserve a facade. Both births were painful, and she had some vaginal discomfort afterwards, but even more traumatic was her anxiety and confusion, her shame at losing control both of herself in the first birth, and her medical attendant in the second. She also shows some effect of her altered role on her feelings.

Mrs C.

Mrs C. a slim fair girl casually dressed in jeans and a cotton shirt, complained of dyspareunia at a family planning clinic. She said that 'She couldn't do it — there was no room'. She was 'stitched up so tight it was painful'. She waited six weeks to have intercourse, because she had read it in a book at the hospital (but she wanted to wait anyway). He was very understanding — 'don't get the hump' — and then she couldn't stretch — he just couldn't get in. Her stomach 'really tightened', she had 'strange feelings' and, although once after a few drinks they had enjoyed it, this had no effect on her idea of herself.

Asked about the birth, she said it was very easy — she had 'done her classes' and it was better than she expected and her husband stayed with her throughout and was present at the birth. She was admitted at 12 p.m. and delivered at 4 a.m. but needed stitches and had to wait until 8 a.m. in the labour ward, for the doctor. She had longed to go to sleep and was very 'cheesed off' and finally her husband had been sent away at 7 a.m. Her stitching was hurtful. When she got back to the ward, it was full of activity and she couldn't sleep until evening.

The same doctor gave all the women an internal before discharge, laughed when they were worried and the woman in the next bed screamed. After her examination she could hardly walk.

At the postnatal by her GP six weeks later she had no discomfort but could not talk to the doctor.

When I asked her to get on the couch for an examination she first closed the window, and then told me that when first married she could not undress in front of her husband. There was no tension or discomfort on examination but when I suggested she examine herself she crossed her arms and blurted out it was 'not nice — masturbation was low'. She sat up in tears, became slightly aggressive and demanded to know what was wrong with her.

She had first had intercourse at 18, premaritally, and with no discomfort, enjoyed a good relationship, although she did find it 'more exciting — more of a gamble' when not on the pill.

At first it appeared that Mrs C.'s dyspareunia was the result of her delayed and traumatic stitching, and the examination in hospital, but it was only on self-examination that more profound difficulties were revealed.

Mrs D.

Mrs D. was a lanky woman in jeans with brown hair and sallow face. She only complained of dyspareunia and a dry vagina when she wanted to conceive again, nearly two years after the birth of her first child. She had had a forceps delivery and intercourse had been painful ever since. She also had discharge and a dry vulva and felt that she had been very damaged by childbirth. Mrs D. had been brought up in a home where any talk of sex was suppressed, and it was only regarded as a duty. Her husband was a schoolmaster who had spent seven years in a seminary before giving up his vocation — only after she came for tretament were they able to discuss sex between themselves. During treatment she revealed that she thought her vagina was a rigid tube that went straight up to the ovaries, and was astonished to discover its elasticity.

Mrs D.'s apparent complaint of dyspareunia and dry vulva, due to a forceps delivery, in fact masked a more deep-seated vaginal fantasy.

Mrs S.

Mrs S. was a girl of 18 who was brought to the clinic by her mother when she had been unable to have intercourse in the 18 months since the birth of her child. She was a large, rather sloppy, pretty girl with long wavy hair. Before conception intercourse was regular and enjoyable but during pregnancy she had not had intercourse because it was painful and now after the baby she had had intercourse three or four times, as a duty, but didn't enjoy it and now refused completely. They lived in one room of her mother-in-law's house and her husband was out with his friends every night.

On examination she lay down, fully dressed, cried, turned to the wall and said her whole body was fat, distended and horrible, and she couldn't touch herself.

Although Mrs S. presented as difficulty after childbirth, the problem had developed immediately after conception. Part of the rejection of sexuality was her anger at the marriage and way of life that had resulted from pregnancy, and a feeling that pregnancy had completely ruined her attractiveness.

Discussion

All these women expressed feelings of bodily damage resulting from pregnancy which had converted a previously satisfactory sexual relationship to one in which there was a complete retreat from sexual activity. In some cases (Mrs C. and Mrs D.) the patient at first focuses her ideas of damage on the vagina and complains of dyspareunia, while Mrs S. feels that the whole of her body has been degraded by

114

childbearing. Mrs W. seems particularly concerned with the way in which her experiences with two difficult births have altered her ability to cope with life and have everything under control. It was only on examination and from their reaction to the suggestion that they touch themselves that the extent of their failure of full sexual acceptance was revealed. We are all familiar with the complete rejection of some non-consummations, and the lesser rejections of frigidity, but these women can accept themselves as lovers and use their sexuality for pleasure, before having children. The stress of childbirth disrupts this superficial adaption and reveals previously masked fantasies or reactivates an early difficulty. Because they were able to enjoy intercourse before this disruption there is often a feeling of desperation about women with this secondary frigidity. They have been inside the garden, but came out and lost the key and are banging on the door to return.

As well as the psychosexual difficulties expressed as a rejection of intercourse, we also see many women who complain of loss of libido in the post-partum period — not a difficulty in intercourse but simply a lack of interest. This is often connected with a woman's over-absorption in her new role of mother, perhaps due to her feeling of inadequacy; her feeling of dullness when confined to the house and nappies and missing her contacts with work and friends; sometimes her mother-hood reinforces her identification with her mother, whose own sexual life she feels was not successful.

One patient, Mrs C., was a Greek girl of only 18 with a child of over a year. She spoke little English and was brought to the clinic by her husband because of complete lack of libido — the only remark she contributed to the discussion was that all her family had married foreign men. Having got her 'man' and escaped from the Greek women's way of life, the care of the baby completely absorbed the attention of this girl.

The cases we have discussed all showed that beneath a tenuous sexual adjustment that permitted a pretty, unblemished girl to enjoy intercourse, there was sometimes a considerable fantasy, sometimes a dislike of the 'messy' side of sex that was reactivated by their experiences of childbirth.

A woman's first step to sexual maturity, her first intercourse, is taken in privacy and we are only consulted, sometimes, when difficulties arise. But the final step, that of childbirth, is supervised, and increasingly institutionalised, by the medical profession. Dr Bischoff (1975) has described the atmosphere of a small French-Canadian hospital — 'open windows and honeysuckle — doucement, madame —poussez. Birth is a fertile thing, hard work — joyous'. We cannot hope for honeysuckle in the NHS but we can give the same attention to the individual's feelings.

The intense individual experience of one can run side by side with the routine of another. We remember the old guide who took us down Tutankamen's tomb, but to him we are one of a host of tourists. So it must be when women are giving birth in a large hospital. If we can be alert to the anxieties and feelings of women in childbirth and respect their individuality, if they can feel that childbirth is a natural process in which they are encouraged to take an active and understanding part, then they can accept themselves as women in the fullest sense.

A case study concerning episiotomy

Barbara Devereux

A GP sent me this lady because she had had an episiotomy and since this and the delivery of the baby she had had a lot of trouble with pain on intercourse, was unhappy and had been initially referred by him to the obstetrician and gynaecologist who had excised the scar and made a nice new one and the pain had persisted. She had been back to the GP and he wrote me a very good letter saying 'I feel that this scar is not due to the actual episiotomy but due to the traumatic process of delivery which she saw as very traumatic'. She came to see me, a young woman of about 30, a graduate. She explained what had happened to her and I said 'Tell me about the delivery of your baby', and she talked for about three quarters of an hour. She unburdened everything. I did examine her as well and she talked even more then. She said how they had hoped it was going to be a really fulfilling experience, herself and her husband, but in fact she had met the witch nurse and the madonna nurse and the delivery had not gone as she had hoped. She had to have forceps, had the episiotomy and subsequently she had not been able to breastfeed. She felt a complete failure as a woman. She talked and talked and at the end she said 'I've never said any of this to anybody. I realise now' — and these were her own words — 'that the scar isn't down there, it's another sort of scar'.

I have heard since from the GP that she did not go back to him for some months and when she did it was because she was planning another pregnancy. I think that really was a success story, but the patient did all the work.

18

Psychosomatic pelvic pain

(i)

Alexandra Tobert

There are patients who present with a physical symptom. Most of these symptoms are gynaecological and the commonest are pelvic pain, dyspareunia, vulval soreness, and menstrual problems. It seems to me that the most helpful way to tackle these symptoms is to say to yourself 'the body is expressing a feeling which the patient can't express more directly, verbally, emotionally'. It is of course a help that very many of these women have already been investigated gynaecologically and are referred by gynaecologists so that their retreat into saying 'Oh, but I know I must have something wrong with me' is partially blocked. They still try to use it but nevertheless you can say 'Well, they did have a good look, let's see whether feelings may be causing your symptoms'. Very often pain is pain in the sense of hurt, disappointment, distress and if one explores symptoms of pelvic pain in those terms it frequently gets better remarkably quickly.

Dyspareunia is often a pain in the area of femininity and one needs to explore it on that basis. Vulval soreness — it is important to think of the word 'sore' as we use it in every-day terms, rather than in physical terms, that is, a mixture of hurt and anger. Interestingly it is sometimes the symptom found in feminist women, the rebels, the ones who had a nice good background against which they are rebelling, but a bit of themselves is pulling them back. I am seeing a pleasant young graduate now who has been sore for a couple of years. She is living with a chap and believes this to be absolutely right and doesn't want to marry him but obviously her mum thinks she should and there is a bit of her that thinks she should too. She is gradually beginning to get in touch with that part of herself but meanwhile her rebellion and her conventionality are in conflict and, in this mixture of hurt and anger against her background, she is sore. Of course these people are treated physically in all sorts of ways and in the end when somebody has used cortisone ointment for two years you wonder what the iatrogenic effect of that is and you have to wean them off it. But again you have to explore what the symptom is telling you and that applies to the whole range of somatic symptoms.

Enigmatic pelvic pain

Margaret Blair

When pelvic pain is largely or wholly psychosomatic it can be demonstrated to be an expression of anxiety, and this anxiety is usually about femininity and feminine functions. The pain is used, consciously or unconsciously as an attention-seeking mechanism to express feelings of: (1) fear and uncertainty; (2) guilt and regret; (3) anger. The most common conditions that these feelings are associated with are (1) menstruation; (2) intercourse; (3) abortion; (4) childbirth and motherhood; (5) hysterectomy.

Puberty with the onset of menstruation is a time of adjustment to developing sexuality and to all its implications. For many this is a natural procedure but for some it is a time of great difficulty and anxiety with a reluctance to accept the feminine role. This can manifest itself in dysmenorrhoea unamenable to prescribed remedies or operative intervention. It can also be a pointer to further problems as many of these patients go on to have trouble with intercourse, difficult pregnancies and labours ending with forceps delivery or Caesarean section. Often this sequence is not predicted but only looked at in retrospect, whereas if the psychological problems of these young patients presenting in their early teens had been looked at, at the time, much of their future pain and trouble might have been prevented.

Non-consummation occurs much less frequently these days but the following case is an example of the use of psychosomatic pain to draw attention to anxieties about intercourse. The patient, aged 22, had been married for three years. She had had a series of minor complaints which gradually became localised to pelvic pain severe enough for her to faint and be sent home from work on several occasions. She was sent to a gynaecological clinic where it became obvious at once that she had severe vaginismus. She would not let anyone near her — the pain was much too severe, even before anyone touched her. She was sent to a psychosexual problem clinic with the message that she would probably need a hymenectomy but it might be worthwhile trying psychological methods first. After much difficulty she did allow examination with one finger and was able to express some of her fantasies and fears. These fantasies were mainly about pain and damage in the form of tearing and splitting. Eventually she was able to examine herself which was a great relief to her. Much later she was able to consummate her marriage and is now considering pregnancy. Most important in the present context is the fact that her pelvic pain served its purpose and has now gone, having been used to call attention to the area of her difficulties which she was unable to express in words.

However, as is to be expected, she still has doubts about her femininity and from time to time has aches and pains in the legs or chest which she presents as doubts about her oral contraception, but she is now able to add 'But I expect it is all due to my problems really, isn't it?'

There are many patients who have been able to allow consummation but then present with dyspareunia. Often these patients are extremely reluctant to admit that the pain can have anything but a physical basis. Their medical advisers, taught to exclude all physical causes before labelling any pain as psychosomatic, collude with the patient, give creams and pessaries, cauterise the cervix, do D & Cs and laparoscopes, and the patient's conviction that there is something physical causing the pain is reinforced. An example of this is a patient who presented with dyspareunia and thought she had something inside her causing the pain which she felt in her vagina at the time of intercourse. She was investigated and nothing physical was found. She took time to accept that her pain was not physical but psychosomatic, but was eventually able to say that she had a feeling there was something in the way as twice she had thought she was almost reaching an orgasm, but had stopped her husband as she did not know what to expect and expressed the fear that to go on and have an orgasm might make her feel degraded or silly.

In this case the patient was able without very much difficulty to relinquish her pelvic pain which had, as in the first case, served the purpose and had drawn attention to the anxiety which she could not at first express in words — namely, her fear of orgasm.

Unfortunately not all patients are able to accept as readily as this that their pain is not physical.

Patients requesting termination do not usually present with pelvic pain — they present their difficulties in the form of an unwanted pregnancy. That in itself should call attention to their problems, but if these problems as well as those associated with the termination, i.e. the mixed feelings of guilt, relief and regret, are not understood and worked with they may need to develop psychosomatic pelvic pain — and some do this.

The puerperium and the months that follow is another period in the patients' lives in which their femininity is strained. If they are unable to adjust to the role of partner and mother, pelvic pain, often attributed to damage and stitching, is presented and, again, it needs to be understood. It is often an expression of anger and resentment against the partner who is often thought to be getting off too lightly with no added pain, strain and responsibility.

Hysterectomy is for some patients a very painful process as the uterus, apart from being functional, is symbolic and represents a large part of the patient's femininity. She may have had trouble with it for years, pain, bleeding, and a determination and expressed wish to have it all taken away, but when it is taken away the pain persists. She was ambivalent, and taking away the uterus still leaves her with her problem which was her inability to accept her femininity completely. This is what has to be understood and worked with if possible. It is often very difficult to do this and it can be more difficult after hysterectomy than before.

In conclusion, it should always be borne in mind that pelvic pain may be not only physical but psychosomatic and much time can be saved and trouble avoided if both are looked at together. While physical examination and investigations are being carried out, an attempt can be made to look at the patient as a whole and see what she is trying to express by her pain.

Two case studies

Alexandra Tobert

Sally

Sally is a girl of 22, a nurse, who has got prettier as treatment has progressed. She presented with dyspareunia and nausea on intercourse, sometimes actual vomiting, which generally suggests deep trouble. She and her husband had had intercourse premaritally but since their marriage there had been almost none. She came when they had been married about eight months.

The child of two feckless people — I don't think they ever got round to marrying each other — but they kept in some contact with her. From infancy onwards she was in care, from which her mother fished her out at a whim, time and time again, and then she would go back into another children's home. There was always the hope that mother would come one day and mother sometimes did and sometimes didn't. Dad said 'I'll come and take you out on Sunday' and she would put on her best dress and wait at the door and mostly he did not come. She was aware from a very early age that mother was a kind of tart and had lots of men around always. She is not sure whether she actually saw her mother in bed with other men but she probably did. At six she was fostered by a woman who denigrated her mother constantly and said 'You don't want to go out with your mother. You know your mother doesn't love you. You stay here with me', and loved her in a way, but a totally possessive way. Sally became after a time the oldest of a large number of foster children and had to be grown up and sensible, but always longed for a parental home.

At 14, at school, she met her present husband who I think was lifesaving to her. These two came together as children and he has given her unfailing support and love. It became clear very soon that her dyspareunia was the pain that she had had all her life and the nausea was the nausea at her mother's sexuality. She accepted this but to move forward from it was very difficult for her, but gradually she did. Progress has been of a very erratic nature. She came to know as she had never known before, full rich sex. 'It was marvellous', she said, but it would go on for two or three months and then she would lose it again. She has been back with 'I can't bear him to touch me' and sadder than ever because she knows what she is missing. We are still at that stage. The good times have become longer, the sad times do not come as often and are shorter, but they are still there, regrettably. Often they are triggered off by the arrival of mother on the scene. Her husband is a policeman and was on duty that night, and she said to her visiting mother 'Stay with me tonight, I shall be all alone'. The mother said 'No, I must go out for a drink. I'll be back soon'. Came back in due course, drunk, was sick and made a mess in this girl's precious home that she had built up. Mother really messed up her home, her house. Down she plummeted into a bad patch again.

She does not come all that often now. She is a woman who had pulled herself up by her bootlaces and has progressed from her beginnings to her present status — she is a staff nurse, obviously doing extremely well professionally and is in so many ways the salt of the earth, but the early damage was very great.

Jane

Jane is strikingly pretty; tumbling golden curls and brown eyes. Lovely face. She came, referred by her doctor because she is terrified of pregnancy. She does not know what she fears or why. She once came off the pill and sat on the bathroom floor for 24 hours shaking like an aspen leaf, sheer panic, terror, frenzy. She talked a bit about herself and said 'I've always found so many things so difficult. There are so many things that frighten me. Injections terrify me. Going to the doctors and being examined. All sorts of things terrify me'. Again it seemed to me that I could not stay in the present with this patient and so we went back into her early life. She was a pyloric baby who had surgery at about a month old. Her mother's mother had a stroke on the day that she was admitted and died on the day of the operation. One may imagine the great trauma of hospital admission at an early age and a distressed mother afterwards. She says 'It feels as though I am all alone and helpless'. Her mother recently went away to America for a month and Jane sank most tellingly into a deep depression. She said 'A few months ago I wouldn't have known what was the matter with me but now I know that I can't bear to be parted from mother and be grown up and have to do things on my own'.

I do not know whether you call this a psychosexual problem but I believe it is a problem for which our skills eminently fit us and I do not believe any of you would have said 'That's not for me'. I am sure you would not, I am sure you see people like this all the time.

19

Hysterectomy

(i)

Pre-hysterectomy states

Tom Main

I propose to give three case summaries of women discussed in a seminar for general practitioners on psychological aspects of general practice. I met none of the patients myself and the summaries are derived from the seminar transcripts. In each case I have altered sufficient details to prevent identification of the patients.

Case Studies

Case One

The first case is of a woman of 47, a regular patient for 20 years and a fairly frequent complainer for ten. She was a big girl, gaunt and masculine and reminded the doctor of *une vache*. She worked as a foreman packer in a cosmetics factory which largely employs middle-aged women. She was resolute and practical, with a no-nonsense manner and kept the doctor in his place except for bodily complaints. She wanted an explanation for everything and intimidated her doctor with remarks like 'How can you be sure?' and 'Do you think a specialist would help?' and 'They say at work that there's a marvellous woman doctor at Clapham'.

She irritated her doctor and he would angrily reassure her — or rather, protest — that he had everything under control and that there was no need to worry. Over the years of dysmenorrhoea, headaches, backache, fatigue states, sprains and conjunctivitis, neither patient nor doctor were very satisfied with each other.

She had married at 35 and there were no children. The husband was four years younger, a tough-looking ex-Merchant Navy Petty Officer. He drank a bit, looked after their large house and garden, cooked the evening meals and was in and out of casual work. He said people marry too young and have too many children and there's a world population problem isn't there? His mask slipped once when he asked the doctor to cure his baldness and then asked if the doctor could give his wife something to make her more loving. When the doctor tried to pursue this he said he wasn't complaining himself, it was just that he'd like his wife to enjoy life a bit more: 'It's not as if we're youngsters, just that we have a little quarrel now and then'. When pressed he said the last intercourse was on Christmas Eve — eight months ago.

The wife earned good money and occasionally gave him pocket money, but now at 47 she complained of backache and heavy periods. The doctor found no anaemia and that the periods lasted six days. He queried the amount of loss but she told him it was heavy and that two women at work 'had had it all out', and felt fine. Shouldn't she go to hospital?

She agreed to a vaginal examination only when he said he couldn't send her to hospital without it, and she suffered this resentfully. The doctor felt triumphant when he found nothing — only a small uterus — and said firmly that hospital was unnecessary. 'But what about cancer? What about my age? What's causing all this bleeding?' Her bossy critical manner again made the doctor angry and yet afraid lest his diagnosis was wrong. He gave her a prescription and told her to come back.

Over the next six months the battle went on. Bellergal, iron and ergot, progesterone preparations. No use, what next, what about an operation? Once the doctor asked about her sexual life. Trust a man to ask that! What did he expect with her in this state? The deflated doctor retreated, but anticipating her usual routine firmly stated that he had decided to seek a specialist opinion.

His letter to the gynaecologist said he found nothing but could the woman be reassured? Five weeks later came a letter from the hospital telling of a hysterectomy for a benign uterus. Because of her age and her hypochondrical fears it had seemed wise and provided useful prophylaxis for the future. The gynaecologist also hoped this would cure her neurosis. The doctor was furious and felt defeated but comforted himself — Thank God she won't come back.

But she did come back over a year later, with her husband. Taking charge as usual, she complained that he was drinking all day. What about a specialist? The doctor tried to reassert himself as her doctor rather than her slave and asked her about the operation. How was she? 'Oh that! I'm all right, no trouble, but what about him? He needs a specialist.' The husband, cowed and unhappy, when asked what he wanted said 'Well, she might be right, doctor'.

The doctor realised that he and the husband always had one freedom — to do what she wanted — but none other. So the man went to a psychiatrist.

The seminar noted her as an anti-man, anti-sex, anti-feminine woman who hated the femininity in herself and got rid of it as soon as possible.

Case Two

The second case was 42. She looked grotesque, about 60 but dressed as a 17-year-old, mutton dressed as lamb. Two garish, rouged blotches on each cheek-bone, much mascara and heavy eyelashes, red dyed hair, much leg, and a painful red-lipped smile on a thin strained face.

She told her woman doctor about heavy losses and how she ought to have it taken away. The doctor found two small fibroids, not enough to merit hysterectomy. She said to the patient she didn't look very happy. What was the trouble? The patient wept.

It wasn't just the flooding, it was her daughter — 19, on the pill and working for the last year as a hostess in a night club in London. That's when the bleeding had begun. What future did her daughter have? 'You know what I mean, doctor. It's her first time away from home; I'm worried to death'. When she'd warned the daughter to behave they'd had a row and now weren't on speaking terms (more tears). She herself had gone to London but the daughter had told her to mind her own business and was now living with a boy friend. The patient couldn't sleep for thinking about it.

The husband was a night-porter/telephonist at the local hotel but also moonlighted during the day as a window-cleaner and was rarely at home. She wanted to work in the chemist's but now these floodings — how could she without the operation?

The doctor asked about her sex life. She'd never got much out of that side of marriage and anyhow he was on night shift. Her grotesque appearance made the doctor go on. Had sex always been like this? Never any fun in her life? Well, he was a good man, a good provider and she couldn't complain.

Never any fun? There were more important things than that, and anyhow there was far too much sex these days. That was the trouble with Elly. The doctor said did she never remember her own feelings at 19? Had she never had lovely disgraceful wishes herself? Never? Here the patient again burst into tears.

She had lived near an Army camp and at 19 had had a marellous short passionate love affair with a soldier due to go abroad. He had been killed soon after — just as her father had been killed when she was ten (more tears).

She felt that if she had not loved them they might both be alive today: 'I bring bad luck.' She still thought about her soldier but knew it was wrong. The doctor looked at her appearance and said she must still have wishes but seemed to be punishing herself for them. Was she afraid to let herself go in case she lost the man again? And the daughter — wasn't she a bit jealous? She and the doctor discussed her feeling that it was too late for her to start now.

The effect was miraculous. In two months the husband left a bunch of flowers for the doctor. In five months the wife followed, wearing the same clothes and make-up but not now grotesque, simply young, colourful, vivid and alive. She giggled and said she had missed a period — whatever will you think of me doctor?

Labour was uneventful. The daughter looked after her and her baby son during the puerperium, and married her boy friend after a few more months. The husband became a full-time window-cleaner and slept at home at night. The two fibroids are still there. There have been no more floodings.

Case Three

The third case was a good-looking, pink-and-white woman of 43, with a rigid, bossy, aloof manner and many bodily complaints. She had discontentedly changed her doctor a number of times in a search for cures. Over the years she had had an appendicectomy, a laparotomy, had twice been cystoscoped and had had D & Cs. She had regularly been treated for cystitis and had been given various tranquillisers.

Her husband was a well-to-do estate agent, a keen golf-club man, known to have a young mistress; he was rarely at home. On his calls to the house the doctor had met him once — an amusing, bluff man who looked meaningfully at the ceiling above which the bedroom was and said 'Sorry, doc, you know how things are. It's a good life if you don't weaken, mustn't complain.'

There were two sons, both at boarding school. The woman looked after a large, spotless, very proper house and grumbled about the scarcity of good domestic help and the need to cook and how men could never understand the problems a woman had to put up with these days. 'It's all right for you men', etc.

Nothing the doctor could do was any good. He resented her discontents and cold, rather superior demands. He put up with her because she paid him well but he wished she would change her doctor yet again. He felt sorry for himself and sympathised with the husband.

For the past four months she had complained of menorrhagia and now the doctor, noticing her horror at vaginal examination, took stock. There were many things to add up — her discontent with her home, her complaints about her insides, especially her abdomen and vagina and bladder, her general unhappiness with her female social role and her anger at men. He began to stop feeling sorry for himself and her husband and to wonder about her obvious misery, despair, rage and pain at so many aspects of femininity.

He decided to pluck up his courage and have a discussion about such matters. But he was still fearful of her and especially at the idea of enquiring about her sexual life, and so he decided to eliminate any chance of failing to eliminate organic disease.

He rang her up. 'What do you want?' He told her he wanted a specialist opinion before anything else, and got the sharp reply that she fully agreed, but asked if she could go to Harley Street. She was angry when he said he knew the best man, better than she.

He sent her to hospital to a dining friend of his, saying he wanted no action at all, merely an examination to be sure there was no malignancy.

Three weeks later he got a note from the house-surgeon: 'Mrs X. had her hysterectomy on Wednesday and is making an uneventful recovery in a private ward. You will be glad to know there were no signs of malignancy and we are hopeful that the pathology department will confirm this in a day or two.'

The doctor was enraged and rang up his friendly neighbourhood gynaecologist who knew nothing of the letter and remembered only a polite grateful patient. He reassured the GP that he had nothing to worry about but he would look into it. Later he said the registrar had been overawed by the woman's complaints of neglect by the GP, had been over-careful to agree with her need for operation, had written her up and had put the GP's letter at the back of the file.

Conclusion

Gynaecologists are often accused of doing unnecessary hysterectomies and causing post-hysterectomy depressions. No doubt many women's lives are set at naught by this mutilating operation even when it is necessary. But life is never simple.

Due attention should be paid to the way some women use gynaecologists to get rid of what is for them the burden of femininity. Presentations often contain complicated human stories.

124

The need is for skill in assessing the whole woman's life and the pains it contains if we are to illumine what may otherwise be an operation in the dark.

(ii)

Post-operative emotional problems with hysterectomy

Prudence Tunnadine

Hysterectomy is often an essential gynaecological procedure which in rational terms may even seem, to some women, welcome. The freedom it implies from heavy periods or from the fear of further conception helps many feel like 'new women'. Others, even with conscious fears and regrets, may have to accept the procedure for the sake of their continued health.

If, however, the woman or her gynaecologist is unaware of what the loss of her uterus may mean to her in less rational symbolic emotional terms, she may suffer post-operatively from sexual difficulty, depression, or psychosomatic gynaecological symptoms, which if unrecognised as such, can lead only to despair for her, her partner and her medical advisers, since surgically there is no way back.

Physical factors
Before discussing these psychosomatic problems, it is important to stress that even in purely physical terms a woman's sexual sensation may be altered, sometimes to the point of apparent loss of orgasmic capacity, if she is not well counselled pre-operatively. The long-held belief that woman's capacity for orgasm rests solely in the clitoris has been reinforced by the laboratory experiments of Masters & Johnson (1966). These showed that in those circumstances orgasm seemed to be produced *only* by the tugging effect of the thrusting penis upon the supports of the clitoris from within. While this report gave much relief to those couples who had long struggled to achieve direct clitoral stimulation during the act of intercourse itself — for many an awkward, frustrating and now thankfully unnecessary athletic feat — the findings only served to reinforce for others the idea that there is no sensation within the vagina itself. This is in my opinion and experience a complete misapprehension, as is the corollary which Masters & Johnson may or may not have intended to imply — that the activity they measured was the *only* path to female orgasm.

If they did so intend, the proposition is patently ridiculous. What of the orgasm of the adolescent in sleep? What of those who, tragically, can only achieve orgasm by, say, anoxia or drugs or the whipping of another? Further, many women who are fortunate in the matter can identify and describe with accuracy the different trigger areas and touches which lead them to different and quite distinct sensations at orgasm, without any subjective or unconscious prejudices as to which might be 'better'. A woman who comes to hysterectomy is often more likely than most to have a 'full' pelvis, a bulky or low lying uterus. Thus both she and her partner are very likely, without necessarily having been consciously aware of it, to have become accustomed to pressure sensations on the cervix, under the bladder neck, or on the body of the uterus itself (as well as of the sensations of movement against and pressure upon surrounding structures) as an integral part of their mutual orgasmic experience. I have met many previously sexually confident women for whom post-operatively and unwarned, that sensation is found to have 'gone'. Several such have been frigid thereafter until able to understand that relearning with new emphasis upon the remaining external tissues and the entrance muscles is required. I wonder how many in their despair fail to seek such help? Further I have met several for whom the sense of it being 'gone' has affected their partners, who have become impotent thereafter; the devastating shock of the first disappointment resonating with some barely conscious sense that their untrammelled sexuality might cause harm as evidenced by the need for their partner's hysterectomy; the fear of damage to a 'changed' and perhaps symbolically unhealed vagina which physically feels 'different'. For a woman who despite her rational good intentions harbours even slight anxiety that hysterectomy will in some way 'end' a part of her sexuality, such unnecessary shock can lead to despair.

Further, though hysterectomy without removal of both ovaries can of course make no difference for good or ill to the hormone state or to an early onset of the menopause, a number of patients do suffer from transient hot flushes for a short time post-operatively — perhaps because of the necessary manipulation of the ovaries. A woman who similarly fears the 'end' may find her fears unnecessarily confirmed if she is not warned pre-operatively that these flushes may occur, and that they will pass until the menopause comes naturally. Thus many disastrous emotional and sexual crises can be avoided by exploring *before* surgery how far orgasmic sensation has been internal, and by warning if so that relearning may be necessary, and by being warned that any 'menopausal' symptoms are not inevitably final.

Unconscious hazards
What does the loss of her uterus mean to a woman in less conscious terms? In addition to the practical factors mentioned, we need to explore with each individual, preferably before surgery, whether removal of the uterus may represent to her the loss of any part of her emotional and sexual self for which she will need to mourn. Only thus can we avoid incomprehensible loss of sexual enjoyment afterwards leading, sometimes, to despair, to marital difficulty at a time when both need more than ever the assurance of value that perhaps only sexual comfort can give, or to true depression. That which may need facing and 'mourning' in advance will vary from woman to woman, but is often in one of two general areas of her attitude towards her femininity.

The uterus does imply the capacity for motherhood, even for women who rationally would want no more pregancies. Thus specially at risk of post-operative trouble will be those for whom, not necessarily fully consciously, the prime purpose of their drive toward sexual pleasure is related to their capacity for conception or mothering. Roman Catholics, those brought up by idealised 'Yiddisher Mamas' (in whom the Jewish people do not have a monopoly!), women who find truly efficient contraception difficult through their need for a 'sporting chance'; others who have been previously sub-fertile, who have had past terminations or above all lost babies. All these may need to be fully aware of and review consciously their past regrets if the loss of their uterus is not to seem symbolically the loss of the purpose of their womanhood.

Others may feel their uterus represents their womanhood in the sexually-desiring sense. They may then feel with its loss, the loss of the 'bright young thing' within them; that this lively part of themselves is removed with it; that they are now 'old enough to know better', as many such often feel about the natural menopause itself. Thus those at special risk here include those who have begun to lose their own sexual enthusiasm at their children's emerging adolescence (as though it is their turn now), who have felt always that sexiness is really for the young, rather than for mothers, let alone grandmothers. Similarly those husbands who seem youth-orientated — sportsmen or ambitious careerists or those susceptible to dolly-birds — may, at this age when they have their own need for extra sexual reassurance that they are not now on the downhill slope, add to their wives' feelings that with hysterectomy they have become 'old bags'. Both men and women need to be helped to feel at this stage not merely dear old souls, but irresistible! And there are many who quite consciously have decided against motherhood — career girls, lesbians, the mistresses of married men — who are surprised to find themselves in touch with the emotional bit of themselves (buried and denied until now) that would have wished for babies and motherhood; that likes to feel it could if it would; that regrets that termination or that careful pill taking — not rationally but primitively and sadly now that hysterectomy has ensured it is too late. And finally there are those described in Dr Main's paper who come to hysterectomy eagerly, unconsciously impatient to destroy this symbol of their hated and feared femininity — yet who, after its actual removal, solving no emotional problems since no surgical procedure can, find themselves at last face to face with their true angry despairing frigidity, all hope of magic gone, and must then find psychotherapeutic help.

Reviewing these lists, which do include those women more vulnerable to sexual difficulties in general, we may notice how many too are more likely than usual for various practical reasons to come to hysterectomy. Thus the importance of exploring any unconscious hazards before surgery is crucial to the avoidance of psychological and sexual problems afterwards.

(iii)

A cautionary tale

Anne V. Smith

Mrs E. was divorced and remarried. She had three boys (two living with her) and had had a tubal tie and hysterectomy.

Three weeks after registering with me Mrs E. complained of a vaginal discharge which was making her sore and itchy. She was 26 years old but looked much older; unkempt, unattractive and constantly nagging at the two children with her who seemed intent on tearing my room apart. I made the room 'safe' for the boys so that my attention could be focused on the patient. This interest was received with surprise, then aggression when I asked to examine her. She sat up straight and said 'There's no need for that … it's just an infection … I just want the pill things you push up'. I explained my request to examine her and she reluctantly agreed, but as I tried to insert the speculum she violently adducted her knees and raised her hips from the couch. Eventually I was able to complete the examination discovering a monilial infection which explained part but not all of her discomfort. When I said to her 'Is this what you are like with your husband?', tears rolled down her cheeks and she described the pain she had during coitus when her husband tried to enter her vagina, not only when she was having the discharge but ever since her last baby had been born, more than a year before. I, having pushed this lady into examination and into releasing her feelings, terminated the consultation by suggesting an appointment with more time to talk. I was uncomfortable and felt that to talk further then would produce rejection of me akin to her rejection of her husband's penis.

She agreed and one week later, when we talked again, I had lost that intimate glimpse into Mrs E.'s feelings. She produced a standard history:

At 16 years old she had become pregnant and allowed herself to be pressurised into a marriage which failed as soon as the baby was born. After her divorce the husband took custody of the child and she avoided relationships until she was 22 and then had good sex, becoming pregnant again. She feared that it would be OK until the baby came and then fail again, and had become depressed and suicidal. Eventually she had gained courage and told her boy friend of the pregnancy and, to her amazement, he collapsed in tears.

He had thought that he was sterile following mumps with testicular involvement. His joy at being fertile allowed her to enjoy the pregnancy, they married, used sheaths for three years and she then became pregnant again. During this, her third pregnancy, she nagged her husband and doctors for a tubal tie and eventually they agreed. Three days after the birth of her third son she was sterilised. She described her horror when her hospital room-mate's episiotomy burst open. She began to examine herself daily and on returning home was terrified to let her husband penetrate 'in case he ripped her open'. Attempts at coitus produced pain and tension similar to that which I had produced at examination. When her husband did penetrate her she found that she no longer experienced orgasm. Her periods became heavy and irregular. Frequent visits to her GP and gynaecologist followed and eventually she had a D & C. All to no avail. The pill was suggested but she had dismissed this vehemently saying 'Well it would seem a bit daft to take the pill when I have had a tubal tie. If I was going to take the pill perhaps I should not have had the tubal tie done'. Here I felt the full force of her regret at being sterilised. Further menstrual complaints forced the gynaecologist to offer an hysterectomy. Mrs E. was very keen on this she said, but had to nag her husband into giving consent. This had been done six months before and she was amazed to find that her sexual difficulties were worse — there was now pain in her abdomen as well as the vagina on penetration. The round of clinics, doctors, counsellors then began. She was advised to pretend to have orgasms, but convinced neither herself nor her husband. Then the family had moved to Newcastle and here she was.

Mrs E. dolefully described her marriage as 'on the rocks'. Mr E. worked away and weekends at home became a battle even though she planned to be less complaining the 'next time'.

I pointed out her wish to change and wondered if she had any conception of what life was like for her husband. 'If I were him I'd leave and make a new life', she said, but when asked if that was what she wanted she became tender and dewy-eyed saying 'No'. Observing this sudden tenderness I reminded her of the tears Mr E. had shed over the pregnancy and of how that had altered her attitude. She was very thoughtful and then began to sob 'I made him agree to that tubal tie and hysterectomy but I would dearly love to have another of his babies. I was wrong to have those operations and it hurts me so much that I was wrong and now I am punishing us both'. I suggested that she might be able to talk frankly to her husband as she had with me. 'But how can I climax when there is no chance of getting pregnant again?' she said, having discovered for herself through the consultation that good sex for her was getting babies.

Six weeks later Mrs E. arrived in my room looking tidy, attractive and behaving in a pleasant, positive manner to her children. When I remarked how well and happy she looked she said her husband had a job at home now, they had talked — and cried — together and felt that there was now 'a chance of being a family unit once more'. She had come to see me not about herself but about one of the children. In other words 'Thank you doctor. We are now OK. It is none of your business!'

My patient illustrates only too well that sterilisation should never be done during a crisis — and to some women childbirth is a crisis. If this patient had had skilful counselling before her hysterectomy, her problems, though not completely different, might well have been much less severe.

Part VI Men patients

Men found it more difficult to 'own' their sexual problems and use the psychosexual problems clinics when they were first established in the 1960s, but now form about 50 per cent of the case load. The following papers include an examination of the special quality of the doctor-patient relationship with men and a study of a series of cases of impotence, with illustrative case studies. There are also the reports of two research seminars, one on retarded ejaculation and the other on requests for vasectomy.

20

The doctor-patient relation with men

Prudence Tunnadine

In my first 15 years in this work my patients were almost all women. Today men increasingly seek help. How does the approach to the doctor-patient relation apply when a male patient seeks help from a woman doctor for his sexual difficulty? Male doctors in training cannot use the vaginal examination psychosomatically quite as women do. They must allow for the potentially sexual content — between them and the woman patient. We do not find this difficulty with women patients, even with lesbians, with whom I often work gynaecologically and with emotional problems. So what of the situation in reverse?

In the early years I sometimes saw couples, but for a man to come alone was most unusual, and the few that did tended to be unsuitable so that if I failed them, it was with a clear conscience. For those referred to me I was usually the end of the line. They had massive social and personality problems and their desperate doctor or social worker clearly thought 'Ah, here's someone else to try'. Those who sought my help for themselves often seemed to be the metaphorical equivalent of heavy breathers, getting, it seemed some relief or excitement in talking to a woman about such matters. But today, in a case load of six to twelve new patients per week, it is not unusual for one or two to be men coming alone and apparently 'suitable' for psychosexual medicine; namely, otherwise stably functioning people who perceive of their difficulties as sexual even though this may affect or be affected by other facets of their life.

Early on I noticed four general groups of patients which would appear often and seem to have factors in common. Some I seemed to handle well; others not. I wondered why.

The young bearded and bejeaned

I met several young men, aged 19–28, typically for example a schoolmaster or social worker, or someone from a technical college, from warm earthy working-class background where their academic success had been valued. But they seemed alienated from these homes by their very education and articulacy, and were terrified by the sexual challenge of say, their precocious fifth-formers. I seemed to do well with these. They talked and in one or two sessions seemed to make modest steps towards a more mature acceptance of themselves. One made a successful sexual relationship with a girl who mattered to him; one, more negatively, stopped trying to make sexual relationships with girls who didn't matter to him; another merely reported that he had been home for the first time in ages, and had enjoyed unselfconsciously sharing his father's excitement over the football results and treating his parents to a meal, as he put it, of 'pie, peas and chips'. It seemed to me these could use me as a model of someone successful in the academic world of their and their parents' aspirations, but at the same time valuing the simplicity and warmth of their needs for home — the other bits of them, as any good 'mum' should.

The 'past it' syndrome

A number of older men, 55–70, complained of secondary impotence usually following one failure for explicable reasons, and clearly had then come to fear failure itself, and that they were 'too old' to recapture their confidence. The trigger varied but was comprehensible without deep psychological explanation; redundancy, a wife's menopausal tantrums, illness, a friend having a coronary while with his mistress. These men seemed to be able to respond to the idea that a powerful woman/powerful doctor didn't think failure or age were cause for despair. This was not simple reassurance; the precise fear needed to be expressed and accepted. The genital examination was often useful and the real fear sometimes expressed at the dropping of the trousers. One 63 year old said something about his arteries, as I commented that he seemed to be well made with no sign of ageing. I ran my finger down the under surface of his penis and reported no sign of arterial hardening and the penis became a little congested. As our eyes met I was able to add 'and it seems to be in good working order'. He roared with laughter and got better! It was perhaps a sexual transaction but somehow acceptable — and clinically useful. He added, 'I used to be rather proud of it once'. I became increasingly sure there is some kind of moment of truth with men if we listen. I always personally examine men standing up simply because I was taught this was necessary surgically. This has implications worth investigating. A man supine upon a couch is arguably to some extent infantilised in relation to a doctor looming over him. One young hairdresser I was examining for sub-fertility had a large varicocoele; but what he *said* was 'Does size matter doctor?'.

With the next two groups I was unsuccessful and this puzzled me, for I thought I understood them well and they could accept my interpretations, but did not respond to them by getting better!

The ageing trendy

These were a number of men in their mid-thirties, typically working in the media or advertising or PR; apparently sexual lions who had 'swung' with the sixties, flourishing in the attention of the dollies of the Kings Road or Camden Town. Now with a real and earnest life of wife and children and mortgages in the suburbs, they found themselves in some uncertainty with their potency. Clearly they had *needed* the added titillation; had difficulty with 'dull' commitment.

The 'big boys don't cry' syndrome

Here I met men of 45–50, public school, sometimes nanny-reared, successful often in the city, with house and maybe horses in the country, children at boarding school or university, worried perhaps about the state of the national economy, but in fact in difficulty sexually about life stretching ahead with one real demanding woman, other achievements complete. Because of their paralysis by the stiff-upper-lip mores, they had real difficulty in admitting anxiety and were begging me to reassure them that, say, oral sex was all any woman would want, and the demands of these awful insatiable vaginas were unreasonable. I was unable to help this by interpretation of the demands of the doctor-patient relation.

A key case I presented at Dr Main's seminar was a sales manager who ingratiatingly told me about his wonderful wife (who just unfortunately asked too much of him) and with whom I not only got nowhere but disliked! The group tried to identify how I felt about him, and Dr Main suggested 'contempt'. I was shocked that it sounded like this. But on reflection later, I became aware that there was indeed something pretty nasty in the doctor-patient relation and it was not all coming from me. I made myself a new classification for differential diagnosis which served me well for a couple of years. There were men, I felt, who merely feared women and these I enjoyed treating. But others, who *hated* women, I didn't wish to know! When I recognised these unpleasant 'vibes' between us at first interview I made no promises; left it to the patients to call again. They didn't. Or sometimes they came once more to tell me I was no good! I accepted it philosophically!

However one learns something, tardily perhaps, from seminars! I recently met another sales manager who was physically very like the other! He too poured over me a tale of a wonderful wife (who was no use), a wonderful mistress (except that she didn't really love him enough), and a wonderful psychoanalyst who had relaxed him beautifully (except that he took a lot of money and didn't make him better) — interspersed with phrases like 'I know you'd want me to be perfectly frank, doctor'. This time I was able to perceive his real dislike and rage towards me and to recognise his need to present himself politely. I put this to him, wondering why he needed to hide his resentment in this salesman's fashion. He could then speak of his father, who was truly violent, and his mother who was 'marvellous' — but who sneaked to father who then did the beating. We found that he had only been potent with his wife when he was planning to leave her, 'to show her what she'd be missing'. Thus we could relate sex and violence, and he confessed that he'd feared having children in case he had inherited his father's savagery. After this one hour's consultation at the age of 52 he managed intercourse nightly for a week and asked for a sperm count in case he might like to have a child after all. The effect may not last, but it was as magical at the time as interpreting the doctor-patient relation to chronically frigid women can sometimes be.

I want to end by touching on this difficult matter of sexual attraction between doctor and patient. I suspect we all feel it sometimes and we all know doctors aren't supposed to feel that, so we find our own ways of brushing it under the carpet. The most dangerous perhaps is that moment in treating a couple when a meeting of eyes with the husband conveys the idea that we'd understand him better than this awful wife. This is not to be indulged, of course, but must not be ignored as a clinical finding. I have thought about this in my anxiety for ethical behaviour and reflect that in real life attraction does usually take two. Only the very immature feel it as uninvited fantasy. Frank Sinatra clearly doesn't care what he does to *me*; but surely he knows what he *does*? I hope we shall learn to use this to good clinical purpose — for not all patients make us feel like this. Again the key case for me was presented in a seminar and I hope I have learned from it — though sadly too late to help the patient concerned.

This was a man whose career as a performer I had followed, without knowing him personally, for some 20 years. So I knew when he walked in the door that I was half in love with his public 'folk hero' image and I was honest about it with him at once. This honesty led for three sessions, even though I had to chase him, to a doctor-patient relationship which was 'good'; not in the sense of all sweetness and light, but frank enough to explore together not only his shyness and fear of failure and of uncontrolled aggression, but also the tough awkward ways he used to deal with women who made demands upon him.

The expectation of genital examination was always there and I worried long and hard how to make it not sexy! When the moment came the tension and embarrassment were there, despite my need to reassure him that nurses did these things all the time! He fled, and I let him, and I still feel sad at my failure to deal with this with clinical skill. But what he *said* were two things. First, 'If anyone offered to masturbate me now I'd fear failure again' (this was *not* of course what I had offered, just presumably what it felt like to him!); and then, 'My trouble is that I had to take my father's place with my mother'.

The seminar asked how I felt towards him and I said 'Motherly' — hastily! The group recognised at once that it was not quite as simple as that. Hindsight suggests that this man's problem — that these two kinds of loving, sexual and filial, can never mix — was demonstrated at that difficult moment under my nose. With more skill I might have shown him that the two *can* sometimes meet — *if* I had not been so worried that *I* might make a fool of myself.

It is something we may all perhaps need to study if we are to learn to make skilled clinical use of any doctor-patient relationship with men.

21

Impotence

(i)

Fifty cases

'I'm impotent, can you give me some pills?'

Jane Berry and Jessie Yorston

In this paper we want to try to show you some work done with male impotent patients by two female doctors trained in the Institute of Psychosexual Medicine seminars and working in NHS psychosexual clinics in the provinces.

In order to gain more understanding of our work by a critical assessment of it we decided to study 50 consecutive referrals of men with the label of impotence given by the referring doctor. We have recognised that the nature of the demands made on us by the referring doctor has a significant influence on our approach to the patients. Most of the referrals were from general practitioners (38) and the remainder were from family planning doctors and psychiatrists.

On the whole the referring doctors had excluded obvious causes such as drug side-effects, alcohol and physical illness, but we had to decide at our initial interview whether the case lay within our scope. We would define a patient as being within our scope when the sexual difficulty is perceived as such by the patient who is otherwise functioning well and stably in other aspects of his life. That is, we would exclude those with significant psychiatric disorder such as psychosis or a profound personality problem. If we decide that the case is not within our scope, appropriate referral is made.

Before we look in some detail at cases and the groupings which have emerged, I would like to share our thoughts about the doctor-patient relationship when the doctor is female and the patient an impotent male.

Many frankly silly things have been written about this particular doctor-patient relationship, and we found that there was a surprising failure to understand that there may be special therapeutic possibilities in the female doctor-male patient relationship. Perhaps we may at present not understand enough about this and its therapeutic use, but we must be prepared to study our work with male patients without being hesitant or apologetic about it. Some of the attitudes that we have adopted in the past about our work with men have perhaps been a reflection of the anxiety and discomfort in the relationship. It certainly can be very uncomfortable!

The atmosphere at the first meeting of the female doctor and the male patient can be extremely fraught and uncomfortable. We have noticed that there is sometimes tremendous, almost palpable anxiety, which can easily overwhelm the doctor. We feel under a lot of pressure to resolve the anxiety — to make the atmosphere of the consultation more comfortable, and to do it quickly, especially when the patient has said in a horrified voice 'I didn't know it was going to be a woman doctor'. However overwhelming the anxiety, it has to be accepted, used and interpreted, not seen as something to be avoided, suppressed or ignored.

It is our impression that those men who radiated the most anxiety in the first consultation were those who subsequently did well. I suppose it is obvious really — they were the less well-defended patients. So, conversely, the lack of anxiety in the first meeting also has significance. When the anxiety lessens, too many men for it just to be coincidence say how much easier it is to talk to a woman about failure with women — because there is no competition. Many comment on how difficult it was to tell their young, male, and obviously virile general practitioner about their failure.

It seems that when the doctor is able to create an atmosphere within which the patient can bring out angry feelings about women, and when the doctor is able to accept these angry feelings and, indeed, gives him permission to be angry, it is therapeutic. It is sometimes difficult not to be frightened and deflected by the anger and antagonism from the man — perhaps because of our feelings of hating to fail to please any man, patient or not! If he is angry and rejecting, it can be felt as a blow to our own femininity and self-esteem — our personal failure. It is even more acutely felt sometimes because of the expectations of the referring doctor, who is usually male, possibly slightly sceptical about our work, and whom one would love to impress! So then — we are painfully aware of our own feelings of hating to fail — how good to be the one who 'fixes him up'.

We are sometimes conscious of feelings of competition with the wife. How easy it would be to 'be the one who understands him when his wife doesn't' — a role traditionally and perhaps best left for barmaids and mistresses!

We have learnt to use our responses to the man — his demeanour, way of dressing, etc. After all, we are not hesitant to admit and use such feelings about women patients.

We note the man who has to try to impress, the man who causes us to think 'How does his wife stand him?', the man who strikes us as obsequious or even cringing, the man who is disappointing and a failure and even the man who is attractive. And yet — all these men elicit feelings that can be recognised as a reflection of something in their own relationship with wives or girl friends.

Some men make us feel dirty when we talk about sex; some make us feel that we must start teaching them, telling them what to do. We've learnt belatedly perhaps to beware of this flight from understanding into instruction.

The use of the genital examination seems to be the therapeutic key with some patients. We experience the same kind of moment of truth during the examination of the male as with female patients. We have lots of unanswered questions about our doctor-patient relationship, for example, how should we handle the situation when the man 'wishes we would see his wife', to instruct her, to tell her what to do? Can we use this therapeutically and indeed see the wife, or is it simply an avoidance of understanding and an escape from the uncomfortable feelings in the doctor-patient relationship?

Above all, we have had difficulty in admitting and using our femininity in the doctor-patient relationship, but have come to realise that this surely is one of the most powerful therapeutic influences — for here is a woman approving and wishing for the patient what he wants for himself, confidence in his masculinity, a good erection and a full sexual life.

We made attempts to generalise from our case studies, and have found that a grouping of common factors emerges. This classification seems to be useful in our routine clinical work with patients, since it gives us clues which can help in beginning to understand the patient's problems. Also it can help to identify a focus for beginning treatment.

So let us turn to these groups now. We recognised four groups — not, of course, with precise boundaries. Patients showing features of more than one group were the rule rather than the exception. We classified the groups thus:

Group 1: Psychosomatic problems with identifiable triggers.
Group 2: Worries about performance/fear of failure.
Group 3: Impotence superimposed upon longstanding relationship problems.
Group 4: Impotence associated with mental and physical illness.

Group 1: Psychosomatic problems with identifiable triggers

Group 1 (a): Fears, fantasies and worries about genitals
  i. Worries relating to, e.g. phimosis, circumcision, testicular atrophy and skin conditions.
  ii. Fantasies of damage due to masturbation.
  iii. Fears of the ageing process.

All of these produced fears, fantasies and worries which resulted in disturbance of potency and loss of the male self-esteem which had previously been invested in erection. A circle of failure was quickly established but we found that these patients were possibly the easiest to help.

Case Studies

Here is a case illustrating worries about genitals.

Mr A.

Mr A. was a 40-year-old teacher of the severely mentally handicapped, referred by his GP who told in his letter of an eight-year history of intermittent impotence and unilateral testicular atrophy which had been investigated and found to be 'not significant'.

He was a tall, thin, tense unappealing man, who made me feel irritated and defensive from the time he sat down and said 'What sort of doctor are you anyway?' He did not seem to need an answer to that question and was soon involved in describing all the difficulties he had with relationships at work with his 12 staff members and how he felt inadequate and not up to his job.

At first he talked just as you might expect a teacher of the mentally handicapped to do — using phrases like 'conditioning' and 'having made a structured attempt to change his behaviour'. I did not get through this defensive remoteness until I asked about his love-making. He then talked of love play before intercourse as 'messing about to get an erection'. He suddenly said 'Of course, we would *never* use oral sex like our farming friends — we don't agree with it — it is all so unhygenic and not aesthetically pleasing'. He went straight on to wonder what part his 'small testicle played in his loss of libido'. At this point I had an almost irresistible impulse to teach him and simply supply information. I didn't, and it seemed the right time to examine him. All was normal apart from the left testicle atrophy described by his GP. The actual examination didn't seem disturbing for him, but straight after that there seemed to be an improvement in the atmosphere of the consultation and he used less psychological jargon. He said he realised that he might have 'taken everything for granted' and 'let it all happen'. He said he had found it difficult at first to talk to a woman doctor but now it seemed to be turning out all right.

On his next visit he was much more relaxed and said he had successful intercourse five or six times since his last visit. He added 'I think I can appreciate women again'. When I tried to appreciate his success, he interrupted me with 'Well, now I can have two ticks in the book'. I leave to your imagination what he thought of the doctor!

Another case illustrates fear of ageing.
Mr B.

Mr B., aged 67, retired oil tanker captain, was referred by his GP with a request for some sort of sexual aid (splint) to help his decreasing erections. He had put considerable pressure on his GP and had previously been referred to a urological surgeon who had prescribed testosterone with no result.

Mr B. was an overweight, well-dressed man with a hearty extrovert manner with which he attempted to conceal his anxieties. He impressed me with his successes as a naval officer in the war. He spoke of having to compete since then with younger men and the importance to him of being successful in such competition. In retirement he continued this element of competition — he told me that he was building a patio which he said 'had to be the biggest and best in the neighbourhood'.

He had had periods of impotence previously under stress conditions but had overcome these and he had enjoyed an active sexual relationship with his wife until his erections had become decreasingly satisfactory over the previous few years. His wife, slightly younger than him, was still orgasmic. We looked at the influence of his wife in the problem, but this did not appear to be so relevant as his own anxiety about ageing and his need still to be young and competent, and we discussed this in some detail.

He departed saying he felt better about the problem and would come again if he needed to. I checked with his GP later and all was well.

Group 1 (b): Contraceptive triggers
    i. Method used — withdrawal, sheath, IUD and cap.
    ii. Post-vasectomy.
    iii. Effect of women who prepare themselves via their contraceptive method, thus demanding excellence from their men.

We were surprised to see this group emerging as an entity, perhaps because in our clinical experience (with women mostly) sexual problems associated with contraception had usually been female. The women who 'prepared themselves' were a particularly striking group.

Case Studies
This case illustrates 'contraceptive triggers'.
Mr C.

Mr C. was 26, a quiet bearded, pipe-smoking market gardener for whom I felt an instant liking. The referral was from a family planning doctor whom his wife had seen for a routine IUD check and to whom she had complained that the marriage had not been consummated.

He told me his story in a quiet, resigned way. They had been married for six months and now there was no physical part to their relationship. The honeymoon had been a failure; his erection 'just went'. He was then able to bring his wife to a climax with his finger — but although he now masturbated successfully two or three times a week, alone, he did not feel able to have any loveplay with his wife. He seemed overwhelmed and yet resigned to the situation.

On his second visit his wife came too and I understood why he was overwhelmed. She was resentful, and self-righteous about his failure — after all, she had done everything and prepared herself with contraception. She had not fancied the pill, but had had an IUD inserted 'in good time for the wedding' and 'even after *that* it was no good'. She had never taken the initiative in love-making — why should she? It was up to him now. I felt angry with her and sympathetic towards him. I tried to illustrate the self-righteous resentment and the pressure to perform and she seemed to realise very quickly that it was not helping and that he needed her participation rather than her contraceptive expectations of his performance.

Next visit they attended together. She was less assertive, and he more assertive. Intercourse had taken place with no problems at all. They did not feel they needed to come back and they didn't. I recently saw them proudly pushing a pram!

Here is another case illustrating the contraceptive trigger.

Mr D.

Mr D. aged 47, a draughtsman, was referred by his GP with recent impotence. He was extremely anxious and said that this was the worst mental anguish he had ever had, and he wanted an injection to remove it as if by magic.

His marriage had lasted 17 years, with no potency problems, but it had been an unhappy relationship and ended in divorce. They had had intercourse regularly but the contraceptive method had been the withdrawal — his wife telling him 'It's you that wants it so you control yourself'. She had been totally unresponsive and eventually rejected his sexual advances altogether. He said 'I had to learn to deliberately put sexual feelings away'.

Now he had met a younger woman who was sexually very responsive, had put herself on the pill and they were planning marriage, but he was partially or totally impotent.

We discussed the pressures put on him in the marriage by the withdrawal method and his controlling and unresponsive wife, and the different pressures put on him now by the expectations of a contraceptively prepared and responsive woman. He returned very enthusiastically better, and asked if I had hypnotised him!

Group 2: Worries about performance/fear of failure
    (a) Problems in a new relationship — beginners, divorcees and widowers.
    (b) Guilt about pleasure for himself ('public schoolboys'!).
    (c) Readjustment after illness/disability.

In all of these sub-groups there was the loss of self-esteem and circle of failure as seen in Group 1.

Case Study

This case illustrates a new 'beginners' relationship.

Mr E.

Mr E. aged 30, manager of a shipping agency, every inch the successful young business man, was at some pains to impress me with his achievements, but he had been married for four months and had been potent on only three occasions. He had gone to his GP with a written précis of his background and problems — set out like a report for a business meeting.

The background was relevant. When he was 15 his father died and he took on the responsibility for mother and three younger siblings. He felt he had to be successful, started a car-washing business and found a job for his mother at his school.

This emphasis on success continued as he grew up. He had several girl friends, but if he became too closely involved and sex was expected, he said 'I became petrified of making a fool of myself', and so he had never had intercourse. When he became engaged to Janice whom he knew to be sexually experienced, he rejected any idea of premarital sex 'In case I might lose her — after all she was at A-level sexually and I was still kindergarten'.

I saw Janice as well. She was also a successful young business woman and there was obviously a big competitive element in their marriage which was brought out into the open. They both became able to recognise each other's fear of failure, and he was soon potent. I see her at the family planning clinic regularly and all is well.

A different case illustrates the pressure of a new relationship involving a widower.
Mr F.

Mr F. was a 53-year-old sheet-metal worker referred by his GP with tremendous anxiety about his problem and about talking to a woman doctor. His wife had died six years previously; they had had a very happy marriage with no sexual problems and he still missed her a great deal. He had had no sexual relationships since, until meeting Mrs M., a widow of 57.

He was impotent with Mrs M. He had always felt that his penis was small but it had not caused anxieties in his marriage and he had never spoken of it to his wife. But he had felt it necessary to tell Mrs M. about his small penis before attempting intercourse with her, which indicated how he felt about the size of her sexual demands on him. I examined him amid his great apprehension and his response to my remarks about his normal penis was of immense relief. I quote: 'I feel a lot better for you having looked at that — it is really normal, isn't it? I'd never have believed that I would let a woman doctor look at me and talk to me like that'.

I saw him twice more. There was no progress with his potency but he seemed to increase in confidence as we talked, and finally he returned to tell me he had broken off the relationship. She had been demanding more than he was prepared to give — he did not feel sufficiently strongly for her and said that talking it over with me had helped him to face up to this.

Was he opting out? Was it a failure? I don't know. Certainly he had still been impotent with Mrs M., but his distress and anxiety had gone and he seemed a happier, more confident man.

Another case illustrates guilt about pleasure.
Mr G.

Mr G. was referred by his GP. A super and attractive young man of 29, studying to be an auctioneer.

Although at first nervous, he soon spoke fairly fluently. He felt he could do without sex for a long time. He had a lot of fears about his performance not coming up to standard and kept asking for reassurance about 'what was the national norm'. He was living with a divorced woman, Hilary, with three children from her first marriage. This was much against his family's wishes; his father, a doctor, had been very anxious for him to conform ever since he left public school and was very disappointed at his present lifestyle.

He could not make love to Hilary and described touching her vulva and vagina as 'awful, just like masturbating'. He described his upbringing as encouraging the 'stiff upper lip and an unemotional attitude to everything.' He'd had a few girl friends but little sexual experience until he met Hilary. We discussed his feelings about masturbating and sexual pleasure and I found myself giving him permission to be more selfish about his sexuality and to think of it as getting pleasure for himself as well trying to please Hilary. He said he was 'amazed' at this and that it had never occurred to him before to take that view.

At the next visit he said that things had been better. He had had intercourse *and* had been able to enjoy it. Unfortunately I was unable to see him again because he had passed his exams and was going to a job in the north of England. He turned up at the clinic together with Hilary to say goodbye, and so that *she* could satisfy her curiosity as to what *I* was like. Needless to say, I did not really like her — in fact I did not think she was good enough for my patient!

Here is a case illustrating readjustment after disability.
Mr H.

Mr H. was a 56-year-old police inspector who received head injuries in a road accident six years previously. He had been in hospital for almost a year and then cared for at home by his wife. He had not been expected to recover, but had made an apparently 'miraculous' recovery. He now worked part time in a clerical job, with residual disabilities of a slight hemiparesis and somewhat slurred speech.

He and his wife attended together at the first appointment. She was overpowering, spoke for him as if he were a child, and was at great pains to explain how good their sex life was before the accident, and how she cared for him at home when 'he hadn't been able to do anything for himself', and how he was 'just like a child'. When explaining that she had done *everything* for him, she talked about helping him with 'pee-pees' and 'number twos'. He sat quietly at her side. When I said I'd like to see him on his own, she seemed relieved.

He came on his own seven times over the next four months. We talked about his new job and his increasing independence and confidence. He had avoided loveplay with his wife, but over the months whilst attending the clinic early morning erections started again (or at least he started to notice them again) and he was able to masturbate successfully. He was very pleased, even elated, with this achievement, but unable to tell his wife.

There was much here to work with and we had established an atmosphere within which we could work, but although I offered interpretations about changing roles in the marriage, his child-like state after the accident, etc., it was all to no avail. He continued to masturbate and be pleased with his erection, but was unable to share any of this with his wife.

Group 3: Impotence superimposed upon longstanding relationship problems
  (a) Dominant wife who is a 'passively aggressive' sexual partner.
  (b) 'Pedestal' wife.
  (c) Premature ejaculation.

In this group we have identified two slightly different types of women involved in the aetiology.

Case Studies
The next case illustrates the passively aggressive partner.
Mr I.

Mr I. was referred by his GP. An attractive, but slightly effeminate man in his early forties. He was very articulate and smooth.

Although at first I found him rather intimidating and felt 'put down', it soon became evident that he needed the doctor's approval and tried to impress me with talk about his wealth and position in the City. He described his fear of being expected to perform, almost like a frigid woman — but he immediately countered this glimpse of painful feelings by telling me that although he could not manage it with his wife, he had no trouble at all making it with casual girl friends in London. In a plaintive way he told me that his wife expected that the erection would be all ready and she would not now take any active part in love-making or touch his penis. He then said he felt he needed a third party to help him talk to his wife and asked if I would see them both. I felt pleased and flattered by this invitation and before I realised what was happening, I had agreed to see them together.

On the second visit he entered the room rather sheepishly in the wake of a bustling woman with bright red hair, whose presence seemed to fill the room. She was indignant and challenging and I was very wary of her. She resented having been brought to the clinic by him. He did not join in the conversation while she poured out her dissatisfaction with his sexual prowess. I tried to point out the resentment and lack of communication between them and explored with her why she could not take the initiative in love-making. I did not get much back from this and was far from hopeful as they left the clinic.

They did return for their third visit and things were better. They had made love and they seemed to be communicating better. She was able to laugh and tell me how angry she had been about coming to the clinic. They said they did not think they needed to attend again now that they were obviously going to be all right and quickly terminated the interview. I felt that all was not really satisfactory and that I had been used to allow them to reach a conditional compromise.

A case illustrates the 'pedestal' wife.
Mr J.

Mr J. was a 43-year-old night porter referred by his GP with low libido but it transpired that he had become impotent. He was a rather flabby, garrulous man who said 'he didn't mind seeing a woman doctor in the slightest'.

He had been married for 22 years, and had no sexual problems until ten years previously, when he had become decreasingly interested in sex and was now impotent.

He was a chap who had always failed at things and had had a depressive illness from which he had recovered, but he was only just able to keep down his present job of night porter. His wife was a nurse and he was constantly extolling her virtues, how capable she was coping with a job and looking after their own two children, plus four foster children. He added that during his depressive illness she had been 'so good about it all'.

I suggested that she seemed to be up on a pedestal, too difficult to reach, and he was momentarily silenced, then admitted that this was true — he could never really talk to her.

I asked him to bring his wife next time in order to have them both involved on an equal basis. To help his lack of confidence, it seemed a good idea to suggest a structured programme of love-play. Over the next few weeks this helped them to communicate on the same level, not only sexually, but in the rest of their lives. The relationship improved and he became potent.

Group 4: Impotence associated with mental and physical illness
  (a) Mental illness, e.g. psychotic illness, etc.
  (b) Organic causes needing multidisciplinary approaches and maybe definitive treatment such as surgery, e.g. penile deformities, etc.

In this group referral to other specialities is necessary but there may still still be a need to be involved with counselling help to work with the patient's feelings.

Case Study
Here is a case illustrating counselling for impotence with organic causes.
Mr K.

Mr K., a 29-year-old man who had had an abdomino-perineal operation for carcinoma of the colon, had been married for two years and his wife had just had their first baby when his trouble was diagnosed. He was referred to me by the health visitor attending his wife. She had told the health visitor about her distress because her husband had been impotent since the operation four months previously. They had both come to terms with the colostomy but the sex problem was causing friction.

He appeared at the clinic displaying all his anger, resentment and hurt about his operation and demanding immediate answers to his potency problem. Nobody had discussed with him at any time the possibility of post-operative sexual problems. Before seeing him, I had spoken to his surgeon who told me that it had been an extensive resection and although extreme care had been taken to preserve the nerve supply as far as possible, there was a 50 per cent chance of impotence.

However, having expressed a lot of anger about his cancer, he was able to tell me that he had felt a slight erectile response when trying to masturbate. This was appreciated as a very optimistic sign and within a few weeks they were able to have satisfactory intercourse.

Finally we produced some figures:

Analysis of Fifty Impotent Patients

Age range (21–73 years)

Age	No of patients	Age	No of patients
21–30	6	51–60	10
31–40	12	61–70	4
41–50	17	71–80	1

Sessions	Patients	Sessions	Patients
2	13	6	4
3	12	5	3
4	9	9	1
1	6	15+	2

Outcome

Enthusiastic recovery	20	No improvement	8
Some improvement	14	Defaulted	8

The objective assessment of the outcome of psychosexual counselling is fraught with difficulties, and we make no claims on these figures, but we did make a very genuine attempt to look critically at our own and each other's cases. We reviewed each individual case and in some cases checked with the referring GP about the outcome.

In summary, we found it a valuable exercise to make this critical analysis of 50 of our impotent patients. We learnt by our mistakes; we learnt about our use of the doctor-patient relationship; and we found the groupings that emerged to be of value in dealing with subsequent patients.

===

(ii)

A case study concerning an impotent diabetic
Barbara Devereux

One morning, the clinic secretary said to me 'You've got a challenge this morning! We've had a letter from a man of 61, he's a diabetic and he's been referred to us by the Pregnancy Advisory Service!' Anyway, I read the letter which had come from the patient; it was not a referral letter.

The man who came in was tall, grey-haired. He sat down and said 'It's very good of you to see me. I feel I must explain how I come to be here'. Rather anxiously he reiterated everything in his letter. He was rather uneasily trying to justify why he was there. He had been a diabetic since his early forties and impotent for the last ten years. His GP at the time told him 'You must be grateful for what you've had. You're 51 now, you keep very well, your diabetes is under control, you ought to settle for that'. I asked 'How did that make you feel?' 'Well, I felt I bet he wouldn't like someone to say that to him at 51 and I didn't feel happy about it. So I raised it again with the consultant whom I went to see later in the hospital in the diabetic clinic and he said "Your diabetes isn't quite as well under control as it usually is when you come to see me; we'll talk about that next time you come." Next time I went there was a young woman secretary with him and I didn't feel I could raise it then and so it got left. I have been reading in some of the journals of the Diabetic Association that it isn't always due to diabetes.' I asked 'What did that make you think?' he replied 'I sometimes get a morning erection and so I thought it must be right that it isn't always due to the diabetes. In the end I decided to write to the Diabetic Association and to the Pregnancy Advisory Services who gave the Diabetic Association a letter saying that there was a clinic where people like this could be seen and that's how I come to be here. I've been impotent for ten years except for one fortnight's holiday that we had in Paris and then inexplicably it seemed to be better.'

I asked a few questions about the fact that he got a morning erection and he also mentioned that he could get an erection with masturbation. He had been married for 36 years, very happily married, he had got a son of 32 and a daughter of 29. I said 'As you are obviously feeling, and I feel, that diabetes isn't going to be the cause of this, can you think of anything that happened ten years ago?' 'No, I've racked my brains and I can't think of anything which happened ten years ago which would have caused a change.' There didn't seem to be anything unhappy about the family situation then. In reply to my 'Tell me about your wife', he said 'We've always been very happily married. I married her when I was in the Army. In fact the Army did me a good turn. I went away from home and I'd never been away from home before. I was an only son and I had always been rather under the thumb of my mother. I went to Germany and I stayed on after the war' — in some capacity still in the Army — 'and I married my wife there. She was German. I don't think I would have ever married had I not been away from home. When I brought her back to the village where we've always lived, I had to stick up for her then.' That made me smile and he smiled too and he realised what he was saying about sticking up for her then. He went on: 'She was fairly well accepted though my mother found it difficult. You see, my father and I were both really under my mother's thumb. She was a little woman and she was known as "poor little Mrs B.", although she was really very powerful. I really felt that it was difficult for her to accept my wife, but she did in the end. There was a good relationship really between my wife and my mother for a while, then my father died first and we helped my mother in her own home at first then she came to live in a room opposite us. My wife resented this a bit but she was very good and used to take meals over. I felt much more responsible for her then.' I asked when she came to live opposite. 'I suppose that was about ten years ago. Do you think that could have had anything to do with it? I did feel rather responsible for her. You've given me a lot to think about and I'm afraid I've done most of the talking.' It was quite true.

At one time he put me in the position of putting my hand up and telling him to 'Listen a minute'; I realised that he had put me into the position of a mother talking to a small boy. By then he had been talking for a long time and I asked him to come back again so that we could go into this further. 'Well, if you think it's a good idea,' he said. To my 'Do you want to come? You don't have to come to please me', he replied 'No, I'd like to'. He came again a fortnight later and said with a little bit more of his blinking and slightly awkward way, 'It's been marvellous. We've had sex nearly every night. My wife initiated it at first but since then it seems to have been marvellous. All has gone all right. I couldn't really think why it was but I felt so elated that it wasn't my diabetes that I felt more of a man and it worked. Once things didn't go quite right, I had premature ejaculation when my wife initiated it, but it didn't seem to matter and we could laugh about it'. I asked 'How do you feel about this?' It was obvious that he was really over the moon but that somehow he had worked it all out for himself: 'I went home and I thought about it and I realised that when mother came to live opposite, you see we used to have intercourse mostly on Saturday and Sunday morning. I'm a printer, I'm still working. I used to lie there thinking "Oh goodness, I shall be late over with mother's breakfast". I suppose my anxiety to please her and to please my wife sort of switched me off.'

I felt that he had really found for himself the reasons for the trouble. He said 'It's amazing, I'm 61 now but I still feel guilty every time we have to go past the nursing home where we had to put mother at the end and where in fact she was for a fortnight five years ago when we went on holiday to Paris. The doctor thought we ought to put her there as it was all becoming too much for us and we ought to have a holiday. I still feel guilty now. Isn't it ridiculous? I wish I had come somewhere like this ten years ago. I wish more people knew about you people'. He expressed a bit of resentment about the other medical people whom heed by his mother and was under her thumb and his wife is still often in charge too. She initiated the first intercourse and looks after his special diet but he had eventually found a woman doctor who was in the sex game and who was saying that sex was OK and for someone of his age. He put me into the position of mother too. He is so much better that I could not help feeling pleased about this, but I am not yet quite satisfied that he has complete insight that his domination is by the mother inside who is still with him, so I am seeing him again.

(iii)

The doctor-patient relationship in a man with recurrent pituitary adenoma

Prudence Tunnadine

In the summer of 1980 I was asked to see just once an Englishman of 36 who had started life as a medical student and was now a successful business man in a trendy and competitive field. He complained of four years of impotence — virtually entire — flagging erections and lack of enthusiasm. When he did get erections they usually failed to suffice to achieve penetration, or he would lose them inside. He had been married for one year to his steady girl friend of nine years. A summary of a letter from one teaching hospital consultant to another reads:

> ... I recently reviewed Mr X. who, as you know, had a bilateral adrenalectomy for Cushings disease in 1965 (at the age of 21). He subsequently developed Nelson's Syndrome; that is an A.C.T.H. producing pituitary tumour. He has had four attempts at hypophysectomy. Following the first operation he also had a course of external irradiation. The situation was temporarily

controlled by the first hypophysectomy but since last year he has had increasing evidence of pressure symptoms with ocular palsies, involvement of the 1st, 5th and 7th cranial nerves and in particular progressive visual loss.

He had very little vision in his left eye and although his vision has been somewhat better in the right, the eye is closed due to third nerve lesion and the vision has recently deteriorated. Radiotherapy has been considered ... etc. etc. Mr X. is worried by the possibility of further radiation doing damage to the optic nerves, but it would seem at present he had little to lose.

I have recently been trying the effect of ... [Here followed a long list of complex new treatments.] The patient is hypopituitary ... I have been trying to maintain his testicular function with injections of H.C.G. but recently testosterone levels are dropping despite this; I am therefore changing this to Sustenol three weekly ...

Lack of libido has been a problem for some time. I am unsure whether this is due to endocrine deficiency or largely psychogenic. The final problem is that he has been diagnosed in the past as having distal ulcerative colitis which has recently flared up under stress ...

That is one kind of report. If I were reporting in an Institute seminar, Dr Main would say 'Now tell us the facts. Let us hear what really happened'. Before doing so I would like to suggest that some readers may have some feelings about this man already, despite the callousness of my report, just as I had some feelings when I was with him, despite the fact that he reported this to me verbatim in the technical language that the report uses and in the unemotional tone of voice which it implies.

So what happened between him and me? For a start the referral was by a colleague who was not his doctor but his friend. They had been at college together and had kept in touch through their common interest which has become my patient's profession. To be asked to see a friend or relation of a colleague is the ultimate compliment and privilege, but it also creates pressure to do one's best, to be clever, to deliver the goods. I felt this about this man even before he arrived and was aware that I do not always do my best work in that situation; I try too hard.

He arrived with apparent confidence. Handsome, big built, well-dressed in a casual style, apart from a devastating squint due to his condition. He sat down and recounted to me this story very much in the way I have just recounted it except that he knew rather more about the technicalities than I did. I sat there listening for perhaps 30 minutes. He sneaked in quite early that he had studied medicine himself a while ago, which I knew; I also knew that he had only completed two years before he became ill. He showed just two flickers of feeling. The only interjections I made were to clarify points of factual interest and one was about his squint. I remarked that it must be lousy for him. He then said, looking down, 'Yes, it's embarrasing. I do work in a world where I sell not only my product but myself in a world of beautiful people and I never know quite what to do about it when I met somebody new'. He and I recognised that he was feeling like that with me at the moment. I also picked up in his factual story that he and his girl friend of nine years had decided to marry one year ago, long after all this disaster, so I asked 'Did you say one year ago?'. He again looked down and said 'Yes. She's a super girl. I don't know how she puts up with it. We've talked, of course, about whether we might ever have children and it didn't seem on; but we did decide to get married. It was a kind of act of faith really'. Then he went back to his spiel about the technicalities. I sat there feeling very intensely more and more desperation, despair, rage at the gods, uselessness, impotence as a doctor. This was so intense and so obvious that I realised that I was flooded with these feelings and that much of them must be coming from him. Thus I was able to recognise that it was a very interesting kind of doctor-patient relation. Here was I filled with all these feelings which came from him; there was he sitting and lecturing me in the language and calm tone of a teaching hospital consultant. All I had to use was this doctor-patient relation. I made some observations about this to him. I spelt out the emotions that I was feeling; that it would be reasonable to expect that he must be feeling many of these; but that he was showing no feeling himself but dealing with it with his high intelligence and technical knowledge. He paused for a moment and said 'Yes, that's me all over. I do don't I'. I said something open ended like 'Well, we all need our survival kit and God knows you must. Is there any special reason, I wonder, why this should be yours?' He replied 'I don't know. I am like it in other things. I always have been'.

He was very interested in the interpretation and thoughtful about it. Then a bit of history flew up, I didn't ask for it. He said 'Of course, I had a rotten childhood. Have you seen that film *Kramer versus Kramer*? That was my story. I had to choose when I was quite young between my mother and father'. He thought a bit longer and said 'I chose my father actually'. He thought a bit longer still and said, ruefully, 'Miserable old sod he turned out to be'. He thought a bit longer. I didn't have any bright interpretations to offer and was still feeling terribly depressed. He said 'I daresay actually that my education was really quite important. I suppose it was part of my way out'.

Now we were ten minutes from time; my desperation was still there as was my impotent sense of longing to provide a solution for him. I said 'I'm sorry I've no magic for you but two things occur to me. One is that it must be awful for a man like you who likes to deal with things with his intelligence and feel in command of himself, to be helpless as you are in the face of this illness; absolutely unable to do anything about it. We do call this sense of helplessness in the face of impossible odds "impotence", particularly when we're talking about impotent rage, do we not?' He was interested in this idea. I said 'The other thing is that erection isn't something you can deal with by intellect or by wishing to. It is likely too that fearing failure to please your much loved wife who has come so far with you is an added pressure on you to succeed. Probably the more you try to think about getting an erection the less it comes up. In that situation this happens to many men'. Up to this point I felt really quite proud of my work despite the fact that I was still filled with my own misery and impotence as well as his. It was time to go and as he got up, having been quite thoughtful; he got himself together again and gave me a kind of a side-swipe; something like 'No suggestions then, doc.' It put me down, and guess what? In self-defence, wanting to give him something, I suggested they read a self-help booklet based on the Masters & Johnson regime. 'It may help reduce your fear of failure and perhaps it will reopen communications.' I was aware that I only give such directive advice when I'm at a loss, but with him I did it just the same.

My normal procedure with patients I am not sure I can help but who are not obviously needing referral elsewhere, is to say 'Make another date. I can always use a cancellation at 48 hours notice if you do not want it'. So off he went. I didn't expect him back, so when the day came and he was a few minutes late and I was sad, but not surprised, I made myself a cup of coffee, lit a cigarette and was starting my phone calls when he bounced in and said 'I'm sorry I'm late. I was delayed at the hospital. My levels are down again and they want to give me some radiation. I had to come and tell you that I don't know how you worked the miracle, but it was a miracle. I went back from you and had the best fuck of my life!'

We tried to puzzle together why and we didn't find a clear answer. I said 'Was it the book?' He said 'No, I hadn't got the book then. I just went home and felt "to hell with it" and it was fantastic. I did get the book actually because you did say so and I thought to myself well, she knows a thing or two. My wife was quite amused by it. But we know all that stuff. You know the world I work in. We were good at it before, I told you, I knew all that stuff'.

Since then, he hasn't been any better but when I wrote to ask after him he phoned enthusiastically, glad I was interested and keen to talk. He said that things hadn't been good; he needed more surgery, more radiation. He was not sure he would agree because he's got precious little vision and he didn't want to lose that entirely. Sexually he had been up and down. He still sometimes had night erections. He said 'When it happens it's a comfort, but of course when I get so depressed we leave it for a while. I can't pretend it's any great shakes'. His parting shot was charming, and in character: 'If there's anything further *I* can do to help *you*, do let me know.'

I see this as an important case for several reasons. First, as regards the chemistry, he makes ACTH-producing tumours since his adrenalectomy so that his prolactin has always been normal. But his testosterone has always been low despite treatment, before, during and after our brief encounter. Despite my belief in psychosomatics, that it should suddenly give enough surge on that particular day of our meeting seems too great a coincidence, so I think we can regard this as irrelevant to the effect of our consultation.

Second, we may notice that the nature of my interpretation was simply about what sort of a patient he was being, what sort of a doctor I was feeling. It was not necessary to speculate as to whether he was showing me the way a man relates to a woman, or a young man to an authority figure, or a son to a mother. He was being a unique kind of patient and invoking feelings in me as a unique kind of doctor and that was the only level of interpretation which was required.

Third, the history that he threw up was in response to that limited interpretation of the doctor-patient relation. It was his association of his choosing, not invited. Had I asked questions about his history, he might have responded with an answer to what *I* was interested in, which might not have been as precisely relevant as what he had to say spontaneously. It seems to me in this context, not so much that history is bunk, but that our compulsion to ask questions about history is bunk, and can actually get in the way of our understanding. For example, if I was to survey the last 100 impotent men I had seen, I think that a fairly high percentage would have given me a history that they saw their maternal figures as bossy and powerful and they saw their paternal figures as shadowy or shaky, so that they hadn't had a very good model of how to deal with women like that.

That is one way of studying patients. Another way of eliciting the same information is that in my presence, or even before they meet me, they are reminded of what it feels like to be that anxious chap — 30-year-old chap, 16-year-old, five-year-old in memory perhaps — confronting a bossy, powerful woman without the support of a potent male figure either at his shoulder or inside his head to help him deal with it — with me. In that light, how they deal with us as patient/doctor gives a precise reflection of the way this chap deals with this situation. We don't have to spend very much time asking what actually happened when he was five or ten or sixteen. Even if we did, we can do nothing to change the parents or the past; we can perhaps enlighten the patient about his present difficulties.

Finally, if we can make such diagnostic perceptions of our relationship with men patients, we are arguably seeing a direct reflection of each patient's attitudes in a heterosexual relationship.

At a recent conference we heard that anyone who tried to treat impotence without getting the prolactin levels checked could be accused of negligence. I don't *always* check the prolactins because nearly all the impotent men I see get night erections or wake with them. It is only when they become aware and awake enough to start wondering what they are going to do with it that they run into trouble, so that one can assume there is no physical cause.

I propose therefore that anyone who attempts to treat a patient, however desperately ill, without examining the emotional human factors might also be accused of negligence.

22
Retarded ejaculation

'I need help — I can't ejaculate —
I'm surprised — I've always been good
at everything else'

Rosemarie Lincoln and Robina Thexton

Case Study

Mr A., a company secretary, made himself an appointment at the psychosexual session attached to the family planning clinic where his wife had obtained the pill six months before their recent wedding. He was 26 years old, had short dark hair and wore a neat, navy, polo-necked sweater.

He said 'I need help, I can't ejaculate. I've always been good at everything, especially sport, and I'm so surprised I can't do this'. His GP, he told me, had referred him to a psychiatrist, but after two visits, the psychiatrist had said 'I can't help you'. He had gone back to his GP and demanded another referral. The GP suggested the family planning clinic.

I asked him to tell me about himself. He talked about his mother, his younger brother who was bookish and stayed indoors a lot, and some previous girl friends. He was dismissive of my comments. When I was referring to his mother he said 'You are implying that I had a bad relationship with her — that's wrong. You won't get anything out of that!' Another time he said 'I think you are talking a lot of *rot!*'.

I was aware he was making me very uncomfortable and was also talking about his wife as if she were not there. She looked embarrassed and I suggested she might like to leave us to it.

As soon as she had gone out he said he was even more worried about his inability to urinate in public lavatories unless he was on his own. It began when he was 14 years old and was most inconvenient in his business life. He attended board meetings, drank a lot of coffee, but when at 11 o'clock all the men went to the lavatory, he had to wait until it was empty before *he* could urinate. He had never told anyone about this, not even his brother, who might have told his mother and she would have thought him silly.

Now he was raising my hopes of helping him. He had never trusted anyone with this information before. I could imagine him, as a small boy, feeling humiliated by his mother standing over him as he used his pot.

He had never felt like masturbating, but had had nocturnal emissions during dreams of intercourse with a woman. This was far more exciting than intercourse with his wife. He naïvely said that the bed clothes must rub a lot for him to reach that peak of excitement. I did not let him see that I thought this was nonsense. Now I looked upon him as a naïve boy. I said he *was* able to share these secret things here, though he could not in the past to his mother, in case she scorned him. I said he had not given me much information that I could use to help him and his whole attitude was that I *was not* good enough to help. He apologised a bit and said he wanted to come again.

His second appointment was more comfortable for me and I said so. I examined him. He was normal and expressed no feelings about me doing so. He talked about his wife and their attempts at having intercourse. She always enjoyed them.

The third time he came in like an excited boy. He said 'I'm delighted to tell you it has happened. My wife came in from her office party and was slightly drunk. She was less inhibited and we made love on the hearth rug'. He had felt less watched by her and had ejaculated unexpectedly and was *so* pleased.

I said 'It seems you want me to congratulate you'. I made a comment about his feeling less watched by his wife, like a male patient in hospital being left by the nurse for a long time with a bed-pan or bottle, so that he did not feel overlooked as he used it. He said 'I won't come back for two months — like the patient in hospital with the bottle, I'll feel free'.

Now I was aware of not being wanted much.

Two months later he came and said 'It's been all good for the last month. It clicked into place. I read a pornographic American novel which talked about the man "pumping". I realised I did not move in and out during sex, so I started doing it. I suppose I'd have known if I'd ever masturbated'.

Once again I felt put down. He attributed his cure to reading a novel rather than to discussions we had had.

I said 'I think you are telling me you have cured yourself'. He replied 'It *was* a help to come and talk — just kept me sane while I worked it out for myself'. I was given no thanks, but of course my reward was that he was better. I interpreted to him that he had put me down and I could accept it.

The technique was: listening and accepting, interpreting the doctor-patient relationship in which he was dismissive of me. In this way he gained insight about how he related to women.

He inhibited aggressive movement in intercourse but he had been aggressive towards me — I didn't retaliate but interpreted this. He realised he had been oblivious of any feelings his wife had had and that he needed to feel free of supervision.

He came early in his marriage, owned the problem; had not thought about having a baby yet; he just sought pleasure. He put me in my place and ceased to feel watched, and, in this new freedom, had experimented and found out what he could do. The psychiatrist who saw him twice may have taken a detailed sexual history — the lack of movement in intercourse had not come to light then either.

At the time when Mr A. made his first appointment, a two-year research seminar was studying the symptom of non-ejaculation as presented to 19 women doctors working in the field of contraception and sexual medicine. We were led by Dr Tom Main. Understanding of the symptom was achieved by case presentation and discussion. Non-ejaculation was defined as 'inability to ejaculate in the vagina'.

Some of the men presenting with this symptom could ejaculate with masturbation, but not in the vagina; some masturbated in different ways using a non-touch technique for instance; one could only ejaculate with oral stimulation; some not at all and one professed he had never even had a nocturnal emission.

The 22 cases studied were referred by: general practitioners (5); subfertility clinics (5); family planning clinics (3); gynaecology departments (3); STD department (1); college medical officer (1); press (1); self referred (3).

Excluded from the study was any man where non-ejaculation was only one symptom in a severe general psychopathology and in none of the cases included could the symptom be attributed to physical illness or drugs.

The doctors, using the active listening technique first described by Michael Balint, conducted unstructured interviews, avoided direct questioning and listened for unconscious fears and fantasies. The doctor studied the here-and-now feelings between herself and the patient in order to gain and offer insights. The response of the patient during genital examination or at the suggestion of it was used a possible clue to the truth.

152

Two groups emerged:

Group A (12 men)
They were actively seeking the pleasure of orgasm for themselves and went to great lengths to find help, consulting first: urogenital departments, ministers of religion, marriage guidance counsellors and general practitioners.

Mr A. was in Group A — he had been to his GP twice and to the family planning clinic four times.

Group B (10 men)
They were pushed into coming by their wives, seven of whom desperately wanted a baby. They said things like 'I can't satisfy my wife' rather than 'I want pleasure for myself'. These wives did most of the talking and demanded that their husbands be made to ejaculate. Their concern was for fertility not pleasure.

The 'old rocker' was one of those in Group B.

Case Study

The old rocker

This man, aged 30 and unemployed, was sent by the gynaecologist who treated his wife for infertility, and discovered that he did not ejaculate during intercourse.

He came obediently, nervous and stammering, a large, scruffy, pudgy man. His wife, dowdy and talkative, said that he never reached orgasm, but became bored and exhausted, while she enjoyed several climaxes. They both blamed his domineering mother, and said that father had left quite early in the marriage, because she was so impossible. His father having left home early in this man's life, had therefore left him unsupported against the powerful mother. He expressed feelings of inferiority to his much more successful older brother who had become a diplomat, but his rivalry was not overt.

The doctor noticed that in the presence of his wife, this man remained almost silent, and only responded when directly asked questions. In the presence of powerful woman he was apparently passive. This patient was asked to come on his own to the next visit, which he submissively did, requesting immediately to break the rules and smoke. Now the atmosphere of the consultation was different, and he gave a lively picture of how he had only once ejaculated in the vagina of a 'bird' he had taken for a motor-bike ride with a gang, and 'laid'. The girl was under 16, and had told her mother and the police had investigated it. He enjoyed telling the doctor of his exploits, and in fact, gave quite an interesting and stimulating account. He related also how he had been engaged to a girl who was an epileptic, but had broken off the engagement with passive compliance to his mother's wishes because she disapproved. His masturbatory fantasies were quite exciting, and involved having intercourse with a black woman from behind; he openly stated that masturbation was much more exciting than intercourse with his wife. He described how intercourse felt like having a 'yoke on his shoulders'. He told of how he had encouraged his wife to wear black undies to turn him on, and then told her he did not find that it did so, and his wife was left depressed and resentful. He had been in the Army, and learned to torment his sergeants, deflating their commands by passivity and by laughing at them. It was a defence of 'dumb insolence'! He presented to them a manner of false deference, but *he* had the trump card, with the sergeants, as with his wife, who also found that he laughed at her when she got angry.

His wife was a religious woman, and a teacher of handicapped children, and he told the doctor that he felt sometimes as though he were another handicapped child (incidentally he often behaved like one). He was ambivalent about having a baby, although highly delighted when he found that his sperm count was normal. He was certainly unsure about whether he was ready for fatherhood and his hobby was making doll's houses for his own pleasure. Characteristic and highly significant were the early excitement and enthusiasm, but the hopes and expectations of the doctor and wife were unfulfilled.

His job record was unsatisfactory. He made poor relationships with his employers. In his relationship with the doctor, he behaved in characteristic fashion, giving teasing, interesting information, arousing optimism, but actually making no changes in attitude or behaviour. He soon moved away and was lost to follow-up.

The characteristics of this patient are those of Group B, in that he was sent by the gynaecologist to achieve a baby for his wife. He was dominated by his mother and unsupported by his father, preferred masturbation, and was ingratiating to the woman doctor, who felt sorry for him, and his defence was passive aggression, that is to say 'dumb insolence'!

The 22 men in Groups A and B had many characteristics in common:

Wife-patient relationship. The men could maintain erections in long and active intercourse, but tended to become bored eventually. The wives were sexually responsive and most had no difficulty with orgasm early in marriage. One man reported his wife having said 'He is a super lover'. Eventually the wives began to feel that something was not quite right: 'He doesn't seem to be making love to *me*. He does it as a chore.'

They wanted their partner to find pleasure in *them*, and wanted the sperm for their personal pleasure in it, and also for the chance it gave them to conceive. A number had resorted to practising artificial insemination by husband.

The unconscious hostility behind the non-ejaculation of these dutiful but thwarting husbands became evident only gradually to this group of women doctors. We recognised the inhibition of honest aggression. One man was described as 'pulling his punches'.

Parents and babies. A few spoke openly of their distaste for fatherhood, but some only showed this in a covert way, like the one who said 'Of course I want a baby, but it will have to sleep in our small spare room and that is where I keep my train set'.

They reported their own fathers as being shadowy figures who had left the mother or had died when they were young or been away in the war. These men were unable to identify with their own fathers, and thus advance their own role from mother's son to father. This was unconscious. In some cases the non-ejaculation only started when the wife came off the pill, or at the fertile time of the month.

The men saw their *mother* as unappreciative of their wish to be valued by her; requiring them to adapt to *her* wishes and orders. They placated her but their obedience was resentful.

Twinning and sibling rivalry. An unexpected finding was that seven of these 22 men were born as a twin. The present incidence of multiple pregnancy is artificially inflated by the successful treatment of infertility. In the early 1940s however, there were 244 live offspring who were twins for every 10,000 of all live births. Our statistician worked out that seven out of 22 was 13 times the national average.

All but two of those *not* born as a twin had brothers and sisters of whom they had been jealous. In order to gain maternal approval when young, they had hidden their resentment about their rival and had sought to be good appeasing children, but had never felt they could please their mothers enough because she seemed to love the rival as well.

It left them *not* valuing themselves. Sometimes their need to be the wives' one and only was made very clear: 'I don't want to share my wife with a baby'.

Doctor-patient relationship. These men presented themselves as agreeable and collaborative with the doctor, so she had high hopes of helping them to be able to ejaculate. As time went by, the doctor, like the wife, began to feel frustrated. Their potency was in raising expectations and then frustrating us.

Other interests. Some of the 22 were keen on good clean healthy sports like football or on solitary sports (fossil hunting and gliding) or sports which took them out at night (coarse fishing). Four were keen church workers. These activities were enjoyed more than time with their wives.

Genital examination. These patients took off some of their defences as they took off their clothes and expressed their fears: 'It looks smaller today'. One could not look at his genitals in a mirror, and when he could only look down, his penis did look smaller.

One almost fainted with anxiety when the doctor put her hand to touch. Another revealed his castration fear of damage to the glans if it were rammed into a vaginal spasm.

Two had bed-wetting problems as children and two were unable now to urinate in public lavatories if they were not alone.

Conclusions

Group A. These men cured themselves in two to six sessions. They gave the woman doctor no credit for the improvement. She had accepted and interpreted their need to stop appeasing women and gain their own prowess. She respected, listened to and understood what the men had to offer. She resisted the collusive temptation to *tell* them what to do.

Important was interpretation of events in the doctor-patient relationship as they occurred. The doctor learnt to tolerate, as a mother would a son *his* pride in his own achievement — his selfish *lack* of appreciation of her help. She acted as a humble co-worker *with* the patient, rather than as an all-knowing doctor whose delight is an obedient grateful patient.

Group B. These men did not improve. They dropped out of treatment. Their initial co-operation turned out to be mere obedience of a passive kind, hiding grudges, fears and hostility. Their intercourse was more apparent than real, whether sexual, social or medical.

These men *were* troubled in themselves, and might have been accessible to therapy, but for the fact they had not sought it and did not want it for themselves.

The absence of motivation in *this* series was decisive.

The way the doctor is approached allows an early assessment of the prognosis. But, funnily enough, Group B, with their capacity to give great initial satisfaction to women, can *still* raise our hopes of treating them successfully even though we are now alert to the significance of this doctor-patient interaction. This is a humbling route by which to arrive at poor prognosis.

23

Personal recollections of the vasectomy research seminar

'Our family is complete. Will sterilisation
mean the end of everything, doctor?'

Prudence Tunnadine

The facts and figures of this study of requests for vasectomy have been ably collated, reported and published by Dr Geraldine Howard (1978, 1979, 1980, 1982) and I do not propose to re-cover that ground. I shall discuss rather that minority of couples who were 'of psychosexual interest', and some of the ideas I acquired about doctoring in dealing with requests for vasectomy.

The structured seminar as a research method
The group consisted of ten doctors with some sophistication in psychosexual medicine and some interest in the topic, and was led by Dr Tom Main. In our pilot study, doctors reported cases of interest or difficulty at random for one term. At the end of this we had noticed enough items of interest to construct a form — not a questionnaire, but one to which doctors must commit their observations in a way that could be analysed for later computer study and, of course, follow up.

We each then reported on the next 20 cases we met, regardless of whether they seemed 'interesting'. One year later we followed them up: first by letter, later, if there was no response, by house visiting. This method therefore collected 200 cases very quickly. It is one any of you who gather together with a common project can use.

The patients
Dr Howard reported that the great majority were realistic happy couples who hoped for no more from vasectomy than it could offer. It would do them no harm, and in so far as anxiety about fertility or contraception was a nuisance, could do them good. But what of those who were less straightforward? Those with whom we learned to be alert for 'psychosexual difficulty'?

First I noticed those couples in whom the man is in charge of contraceptive matters. Using coitus interruptus or french letters, these men are not seen by doctors

156

except in cases of sexual difficulty. Whilst most simply preferred these ways, I learned to be interested in those couples for whom it *had* to be this way. The request for vasectomy was a logical step for some. We are all familiar with those women who have difficulty in contracepting, and whose men thus *must*. But here we met sometimes men who themselves felt they *had* to be in charge; through some difficulty in trusting to their women, or to keep them in their place.

One such was a police sergeant. He controlled the interview by telling the doctor how he had always used withdrawal and was very good at it; they only had, say, six children and a couple of unplanned ones. He was going to have a vasectomy and the doctor was going to sign the form and that was that. His mouselike wife sat dumb and the doctor, thinking she was supposed to be doing a good joint counselling here, had to turn her back on him to ask the wife 'And I wonder how you feel about all this?' As the mouse blinked and made to open her mouth, the man slammed his fist on the desk and shouted 'She thinks it's a good idea!'

More exaggerated forms of the wife who couldn't and the man who must presented; couples who perhaps found each other or created each other or both. They had become castrating women with placating husbands. The angry disappointed women 'wanted him done', but equally the men were determined to get themselves done; sometimes protectively in fearful submission, sometimes in real 'downing tools' passive aggression, inhibiting overt resentment with a kind of tooth-sucking 'right then', as though to say 'that'll show her'. Vasectomy could probably do no harm though it might leave them with their hope of magic gone, their less than conscious marital warfare nakedly revealed. It could certainly do no good.

We also met a phenomenon which Dr Main referred to as 'men's club efficiency', and which I came to think of as the 'Michael Parkinson syndrome'. We met, for example, whole fire stations or cricket clubs in which vasectomy had become the 'in thing'. Here I have learned to watch out for the *one* member for whom it is not such a good idea. Sometimes it is the one who isn't confident enough to resist his peers and be the odd man out, who I think is most likely to do badly. I have met a similar situation which I call the 'chicken' difficulty belonging to this brave new world where husbands are expected to attend childbirth. One recently — having become quite impotent from the birth on — said tearfully of the labour ward 'It was like an abbattoir, doctor', and confessed that as the tough guy of the four-ale bar he simply hadn't dared to say no to attending.

Then there were those who were looking, it seemed, for a 'final solution' — with all the sinister overtones that phrase has. To what? To uncontrolled or disappointing fertility sometimes; sometimes, it seemed, to sexuality or to the fears of its harm. One couple had a disastrous history: they were poor, desperate and had two or three badly damaged children. Vasectomy was realistic; it was clear to a sensitive doctor that their love-life represented a clinging by the finger nails to such happiness as they could salvage. She was aware that the guilt and shame and misery might in other circumstances profit from airing. The pain was too much and too near the surface and the doctor intuitively respected their pitiful defences. They did well. But in another, the transvestite husband seemed to be looking to vasectomy as a kind of self-castrating punishment for his shameful secret. Vasectomy was not recommended and he was referred for psychotherapy. At a less serious level, several wives hoped it might 'cool him down'.

Then we were interested to meet a number of young, childless, sometimes not even yet married or sexually committed youngsters. I came to think of these as the 'escapers' or 'travelling people' (after, I think, a Bob Dylan song around at that hippy time). We were all anxious about these. One was found at follow-up to be no longer with the same member of the commune as he brought to the session. Another couple wrote happily from a tent on the slopes of Mount Kenya. One couple I met were delighted — they had been saving up since their engagement for this. She preferred horses; he was a lone long-distance yachtsman. They went off vasectomised and penniless to New Zealand, holding hands and quite uncomprehending of *my* anxieties! Such patients would present idealistic ideas about the population explosion saying that the world is no place to bring children into unless you are really crazy about them. Yet I have my own reservations about this. I knew one young man who talked this way and who, not to my surprise, came for and got vasectomy, though not from me. His first marriage had failed, his wife taking his one beloved son. I knew that in his own childhood the world had indeed seemed so hostile that to risk having, and perhaps again losing a child he might come to love, was too difficult for him. But he maintained his 'idealism' to the last and got his vasectomy despite the youth and nulliparity of his second wife. When I last heard of them he had persuaded her to join him in his latest hobby, hang-gliding. One can only speculate where his self-destructiveness may lead him — though he can no longer afford the racing cars he drove when I first knew him.

Finally, we had a box on the form for 'overstretched motherhood', an idea which was revealed often and made sense of a number of requests in which the capacity for loving mothering had come to a halt. What was interesting was how this varied in actual quantity — not all these had three or four under-fives. We met it sometimes in mothers of only one, or one and a termination. Perhaps the 'escapers' were exhibiting it with none at all! 'Fatherhood overstretched' was worthy of note too, as well as fear of fatherhood, and again with great variation in actual numerical fathering.

Doctoring problems
As usual in such groups, I felt I learned some technical things which have stayed with me.

Firstly we saw, of course, always couples. Dr Main felt our technique was actually limited by this. I disagreed in that we got a quick appreciation of the marital interaction. But equally it was sometimes difficult to elicit what one partner might feel in the presence of the other. Different doctors found their own ways round this, sometimes, for example taking the opportunity of an individual quiet word when doing the physical examination of each separately. One must emphasise here the importance of examining both. Vasectomy may be foolish for the husband whose 35-year-old multiparous wife has already 14-week-sized fibroids. One teratoma of the testis was found on routine examination of an apparently healthy candidate.

One thing most of us found difficult was a phenomenon that, in the context of the abortion research seminar, we came to call the 'rubber stamp syndrome'. Doctors found themselves variously uneasy or resentful of the situation in which patients seek not help, but a yes or no to their own prescription — in this case, vasectomy. I personally used Dr Michael Courtenay's method to get over the panicky 'fight' inherent in requests for abortion and would say 'Yes, that can be arranged if you're sure it's what you want. Now let's talk about it'. But some of our patients were none too keen to talk about it, and resented having, as they felt, to justify a rational and personal decision.

This leads me to recall the variation in the doctors' attitudes both to vasectomy and to 'meddling'. Many of us were surprised to find ourselves rather against the operation, particular when, as one doctor said, the patient was such a gorgeous man that she felt he should father a thousand children! And we needed sensitivity sometimes to leave well alone, reflecting the feeling of many of us that ultimately it was the patients' decision; that we could only hope to help them make it a more aware and informed one.

The follow-up

This was a trial to many of us who felt intrusive. We felt that the patients had the right to withhold information if they wished. Yet the results were surprisingly complete as a result of the mutual nagging that was necessary, and without it we should have made some false assumptions. I remember three cases in particular.

Case Studies

One doctor reported a Yorkshire miner of West Indian origin who seemed like Muhammed Ali, Harry Belafonte and Sydney Poitier rolled into one! With his three beautiful children and his cuddly local girl wife and an obvious warm relationship they seemed an ideal case for vasectomy. The doctor was therefore devastated to hear at follow-up that he had been impotent, apparently, since the operation. Such was her concern that she made a long and difficult journey to their home. There she found this beautiful hulk hunched in the kitchen surrounded by well-meaning and motherly neighbours in slippers and rollers, his wife out to work because of the three-day week, and his manhood taken from him not by the vasectomy but by the government's difficulties with his trades union. When full-time working resumed and his wife came home, he became master of himself again both in house and bed.

Another was a retired Army officer and his nurse wife. They seemed show-offs when I first met them, protesting too much, it seemed, about the Singapore Swimming Club and the sailing at Kyrenia. I suspected their motives for I knew something of this world and it didn't feel right. At follow-up I visited them in the two-up two-down in the poor area of a town which was all they could afford. He was travelling 50 miles by motor bike in all weathers to the only job he could get. She set off to her night shift as soon as she had fed him and the children. As his kids scrambled over him full of love in front of a sputtering gas fire, their need to remember better times took on a totally different light.

And finally, I remember a teacher who had seemed rather bossy and castrative to her charming husband in the clinic. When followed up at home she was found bedraggled and literally toiling over a hot stove. He was outside tinkering happily with his hobby, fast cars!

Our conclusions

One *bon mot* which was generally agreed was 'Never make permanent decisions in a crisis'. In the context of terminations, deaths of parents or illnesses of children, or infidelities, we found that easy vasectomy was often sought and often unwise.

As a result of this study, we postulated these criteria for a 'good result':

1. A good mutual relationship as revealed to a trained doctor. In one case there were all kinds of horrors in the history, but two skilled doctors agreed 'they thought they were all right'. They were!

2. A good sex life as revealed to a trained doctor. I remember a 'cockney sparrow' couple. They said they had 'worked 'ard for their kids and it was time for some freedom', and when I asked about their love-life he said, as they laughed at each other, 'Well it's smashin', in'it?' — and I might not have been there!

3. Mutuality of request and of contraceptive effort — by which we meant no anxiety in a trained doctor about who is pushing whom to be sterilised.

4. If anxiety is present, that this should be aired and shared *before* the operation.

5. Realism of expectations: that they hope for from the operation, a sperm-free ejaculation — and only that.

Other Settings

Part VII Primary care

The papers in this section are reporting similar problems to those in the previous section, but I have arranged them separately because the emphasis is on the way seminar training has enabled the doctors to have greater insight in their work in a particular setting. The group includes primary care situations both in the community health clinics for family planning and vasectomy counselling and in general practice, as well as 'walk-in' youth advisory clinics for young people. Because it pertains to contraception I have also included Dr Blair's paper on anxieties about the pill. Because many of the doctors in the first seminars worked in the family planning clinics there are, paradoxically, many psychosexual problems clinics, run by the Community Health Service and therefore classified as primary care, which receive referrals from NHS consultants. They are staffed in the main by members of the IPM and many of the findings in the previous section come from work in these clinics.

24

Problems presenting in contraceptive work

'Nothing seems to suit, doctor'

Elphis Christopher

It has become a truism that there is much more to contraception than fitting a coil or prescribing the pill. The doctor who disagrees with this will soon discover the error of his ways. The decision about whether to use contraception at all or which particular method can be an extremely complex one with many factors involved. It is the purpose of this paper to explore some of these factors so that the doctor can deal more sensitively and effectively with his 'difficult' patients — to understand better what the difficulty is about. The doctor faced with a woman (or couple) who cannot make up her mind about which, if any, method to use, or who is full of what may sound like reasonable complaints about the methods, is likely to get frustrated, irritated and even angry, especially if he has a waiting room full of patients. The doctor, in desperation, may attempt to force a decision upon the woman. However, the result of that may well be misuse of the method leading to an unwanted pregnancy, further complaints about the method, or the patient seeking advice elsewhere. The woman who says, almost in the same breath, 'I don't want to get pregnant but I can't take the pill, use the coil, etc.', is making an illogical statement; logically, if she does not want to get pregnant but cannot find a satisfactory method of contraception, she should not have sexual intercourse. However, this is not about logic — it is about ambivalence, uncertainty, wanting two things at once or nothing at all. The indecision is confusing to both the patient and the doctor and the doctor will need to probe beneath the surface of this seemingly contradictory statement. Before looking at this, what might be called the 'reality factors' in contraceptive work need to be explored.

'Reality factors'

It must be remembered that the contraceptive methods have had a very bad press in recent years, every side-effect highlighted and often exaggerated. Reliance is placed on the anecdotal story so that it is made to look as though every woman will die from thrombosis on the pill. In addition to this are the old (and new) wives' tales

163

which circulate: the coil gives you VD, the pill makes you sterile, spermicides give you cancer, the government puts a hole into every tenth sheath to keep the population figures up, sterilisation makes you fat. The injectable contraceptives, particularly depoprovera, have come in for great criticism. It is said to make women sterile, give them cancer, cause their babies to be deformed, make their hair fall out, prevent orgasms and turn women into lesbians! Much of this criticism has been spearheaded (if that is the right word!) by feminist groups, angry and resentful that contraception is left to women but controlled by male doctors. I recently read a 'spoof' scientific paper on a new wonder contraceptive called 'Armpitin'. It had *no* side-effects, carried *no* risk to health or future fertility, did not harm the foetus and was completely and instantaneously reversible. It did not interfere with the sex act and it actually increased libido. It was a chemical (non-toxic, non-allergic) rubbed into the female armpits (hence 'Armpitin') which suppressed spermatogenesis when the male partner sniffed its fragrance, at the same time increasing his desire. What could be better?

We must accept that we do not have the perfect contraceptive (for everyone) — all methods do have side-effects and drawbacks. Heavy, prolonged periods with the coil do restrict lovemaking; coil threads can cause male dyspareunia ('like putting your whatsit in a bed of thorns', as one patient graphically described it); the cap is rather messy; and putting on the sheath does interrupt love-play and male sensation is not as intense. One patient described how he was 'allergic to them rubbers'; he meant he lost his erection. A man has to have confidence in his potency to use the sheath. Anxieties must be listened to and straightforward information given to the patient to enable her to come to her own decision. Having said that, it needs also to be said that most people do settle on a method without too much bother. So what is it that prevents others doing so?

Some factors involved in indecision
Personal conflicts. Some kind of conflict may be going on between what the patient really wants, what she thinks she ought to want and what others think she should do. For example: (a) The woman who would very much like a pregnancy but whose partner is opposed to it, perhaps for good reasons, e.g. financial considerations, will find fault with every method and though claiming that she does not want to get pregnant somehow contrives it. (b) The girl who has not really given herself permission to be involved in a sexual relationship and is uncertain in it may feel that settling on a method of contraception is somehow definitely sanctioning it. Thus by not using contraception, as no method proves suitable, when sex happens it is not her fault. She did not consciously intend it.

There may be conflict about taking responsibility for one's behaviour in any sphere, not just the sexual one. To take responsibility means also accepting blame when things go wrong. For some people it is easier to blame others or 'fate' or 'God's will'. Thus, what happens has nothing to do with the individual. Getting pregnant becomes part of this: 'It was meant to be.' As one patient with five children put it, 'If you're meant to have another, then even that pill can't stop you'. If none of the methods is suitable for you then you can hardly be blamed if the inevitable happens. Using contraception and taking control of this area of one's life may threaten the view that one is powerless. Hence there may be a need to render

164

the contraceptive methods 'useless' and ineffective. Doubts and uncertainties about femininity, masculinity, identity and self-value often lead to an inability to settle on a method, or complaints. Some women can only see themselves as mothers, not as individuals. The role of mother carries respectability and value. This applies equally to some men who see their potency and virility bound up with how many children they produce. Women who see themselves solely as mothers sometimes dispense with men once they have been impregnated, believing that children are a woman's concern and cannot be shared. These are the women who, when asked what they are going to do about contraception, respond that they 'do not want anything as they are not doing anything' which is often true until they want the next child. Such women are often almost pathologically concerned about the effect of the methods on their fertility which is often their only perceived asset. Thus they may make statements such as 'The coil blocks your tubes' and 'The pill makes your babies abnormal'.

Case Study

Ann

Ann was single, 28, with seven children by almost as many partners. She found fault with all the methods — she had 'fallen' on the pill, the coils had dropped out, the cap was too fiddly and her men did not like sheaths and neither did she. She refused the offer of sterilisation as she had heard that it made your periods heavy. Ann's role as a mother was constantly undermined by her own mother, now past the menopause and unable to have any more children of her own. She lived nearby and had always made Ann feel useless and once the babies became toddlers she somehow 'appropriated' them. Ann felt empty and lost without a baby in her arms. Indeed, she always looked marvellous when pregnant and had easy births. After much social work support and rehousing away from mother, she accepted sterilisation after her eighth child (and twelfth pregnancy) by a different partner. Sadly, the Anns of this world are frequently poor or indifferent parents who neglect or injure their children, who may then have to be taken 'into care'. The feelings of failure and loss become too unbearable and the woman becomes pregnant again to replace the child who is gone.

Rivalling mother or a sibling or in-law or a desperate need for a boy when all the other children are girls (or vice versa) can also result in the woman finding fault with every method until she has achieved her desired end, e.g. having more children than mother.

The search for identity and self-esteem and seeking the solution in motherhood is seen in some teenagers, particularly those who are less able. Such girls, who may also be 'in care' of the local authority, are often brought to clinics for contraception by their social worker, understandably worried because they are 'at risk'. The girl may agree to take the pill but is full of complaints about it when she returns to the clinic. The girl may well be following the pattern set by her own mother whose power comes from having babies. Such girls often resent being controlled in any way, so being defiant and critical about contraception is another way of cocking a snook against authority. They sometimes say contraception is akin to murder.

Conflicts about the future and the woman's role can lead to fault-finding with and ambivalence about contraception after successful use. This is found nowadays with some successful career women in their early to mid thirties, 'spoiled' in some ways by the pill which has allowed them to pursue both their career and a sexual relationship free from the fear of pregnancy; they begin to feel that time is running out and that they ought to make a decision about whether or not to have a child before it is too late. However, they also realise that a child will probably mean a change in their career plans, hence the ambivalence. Such women suddenly decide that it is dangerous to remain on the pill (they may bring articles to the doctor, on the pill and its dangers); fitted with a coil, they claim it is causing discomfort; the cap and sheath are 'too much bother'. Interjected between these complaints, anxieties about pregnancy are expressed: 'Am I too old to have a baby?', 'Will it be normal at my age?', 'I wonder if I'm still fertile after all these years on the pill'. Sometimes proof of fertility is all that is required.

Case Study
Miss B.

Miss B. was a highly successful editor of 32 with a publishing firm. She had taken the pill without any problems for seven years. She suddenly began to complain of lack of interest in sex, was tired, had no energy, etc. Although she was adamant (perhaps too much so?) that she did not want to be pregnant, she felt she should stop the pill and try the coil. After two months she requested removal of the coil because it was painful.

As the cap was 'too much bother' she decided to try a 'natural' method as she had read about it somewhere. When she became 'accidentally' pregnant, she was both thrilled and horrified. After much agonising she decided on an abortion and returned to the pill.

Conflicts to do with the relationship. The inability to settle on a method or complaints about methods are seen at the beginning and ending of relationships. The uncertainty surrounding the start of a relationship, whether this is really 'the one' again, often means that the woman cannot give herself permission to use contraception. She may feel she is being 'too forward' and that the boy friend will feel that she is trying to tie him down in some way. Hence expressions such as, 'I did not know him well enough to take the pill'. When a relationship is ending (perhaps not fully acknowledged by the partners) the confusion of feelings — anger, disappointment, resentment — can lead to a rejection of the contraception or complaints about the current method. Sometimes the woman stops the pill hoping thereby to indicate to the partner what she cannot put into words, that the relationship is over or that she does not want sex. The quality of a relationship determines whether contraception is used consistently. The kind of relationship in which there is mutual trust and joint decision-making usually poses no problems with contraception. Where the relationship is based on one partner trying to control or manipulate the other, where there is envy and fear of the opposite sex, power battles, insecurity, lack of trust, little discussion, then there will usually be associated problems with contraception even though neither partner wants a pregnancy. The insecure man (afraid of the threat of male rivalry) may try to keep his wife almost constantly pregnant so that she is always busy with the care of children, in an attempt to control her. Such a man will not allow his partner to use contraception and should the woman try to escape his control and use contraception there will be fierce arguments and even violence. The man may well have angry scenes with the doctor and accuse him of forcing his wife to use this 'dangerous' method which will make her ill.

Mrs C.

Mrs C. was 28 years old with four children and had also had three miscarriages. After each delivery contraception was discussed; she found fault with each of the methods. Eventually she decided to try a coil but failed to keep her appointment. After the fourth child her health visitor referred her for domiciliary family planning advice.

Mrs C. was very pleasant and made tea for the doctor and decided she would take the mini-pill, though was not too keen. A phone message from the health visitor two weeks later revealed that Mrs C. was not taking the pill. At the doctor's second visit Mrs C. was out taking the children to school, but Mr C. was there. He was ingratiating and seemed delighted to hear that his wife had been 'naughty' and had not taken the pill. When asked what he felt he disclaimed all responsibility and said it was up to her. He then said, almost as an aside, that he did not know how the last pregnancy had happened since they had only had sex once so his wife must have chosen the right time. Underneath his ingratiating behaviour the doctor sensed a great deal of anger and indeed this proved to be so. The story which came to be revealed in time was of a marriage where the husband had been autocratic and self-centred, with a clear idea of what a man's role was to be. He did not help his wife or share the care of the children. Repeated arguments led to violence and the wife left, taking the children to a 'battered wives' refuge'. Social workers, etc., were involved, making the husband feel humiliated and resentful. The wife eventually returned on condition that he would change; she refused to have sex with him in order to punish him but 'allowed it' when she wanted to get pregnant. Here we see a 'battle between the sexes' in earnest, each struggling for power with part of the contest taking place in the sexual arena, and the non-use of contraception being used as a weapon and means of control. The situation has been partially resolved by him deciding to use the sheath when she 'lets him' have sex!

Power battles can also take place between partners who cannot resolve which partner should use contraception. The man who refuses to use the sheath places the responsibility for contraception on the woman. She may feel that if he really cared about her he would not want her to risk her health with the pill or coil. Resentment may then take over with the woman unable to decide on a method, or full of complaints with the one she decides to use. Interestingly, wives whose husbands practise coitus interruptus often say in response to the question 'What are you doing about contraception?', 'My husband takes care of me'.

Conflicts to do with sex and sexual relationship. Some couples feel that sexual intercourse is a natural, spontaneous act which cannot be planned for: pleasure must not be anticipated. Thus, premeditation of any kind — and hence birth control — is unnatural, against nature. This view is often held by 'romantics' whose concept of and need for the 'perfect sex act' has more to do with fantasy than reality. These are sometimes the same people who are fastidious and cannot tolerate the 'mess' of sex, particularly vaginal fluid and semen. Their concept of the sex act is one performed by pure angels with dry thighs who always look beautiful. Eventually, the 'naturalness' of repeated pregnancy becomes too burdensome and a contraceptive method is usually settled on.

Such couples need to confront the gap between fantasy and reality. Some women strongly believe that sex is solely for procreation and not for pleasure, which is incidental and tends to be a male prerogative. Once the woman has the number of children she can cope with she is faced with a painful choice; not enjoying the sex act herself she cannot see why she should put up with the side-effects or inconvenience of contraception since 'he's the one that gets the pleasure'. By not using contraception, or finding fault with each method, she hopes to control or moderate her partner's sexual advances by using the fear of an unwanted pregnancy. Sex for pleasure can be seen by such women as morally degrading, reducing them to the level of prostitutes used for convenience. These are the women who say proudly, 'Sex is no bother to me', and expect to be congratulated on their virtue. The doctor may come in for the same treatment as the partner. References are made to 'your difficult job', and 'I don't know how you do it', indicating disgust with the doctor who has too much interest in sexual matters for his own good! When these women become pregnant again they can put the blame onto their partner; it had nothing to do with them, they did not want sex in the first place. It becomes a case of 'cutting off your nose to spite your face'.

Dora was one such, a 36-year-old married woman with six children who found fault with everything and had plausible reasons why she could not use contraception. She felt her husband should 'be done', i.e. have a vasectomy. After all, sex did not bother her — she could do without it. She only did it to satisfy him (and his dirty desires!). Thus, battle went on until Dora had her seventh child. The pregnancy was difficult, ending with a premature baby. She then decided to be fitted with a coil.

Problems with contraception and complaints about the methods may hide a sexual problem. For example, the woman whose partner has premature ejaculation may get so frustrated that sex is over before it has begun that she may decide there is no point in her taking precautions. Unable to complain of her husband's difficulty directly, she may present with complaints about the contraceptive method. The woman or man may only allow themselves to become sexually excited when there is a risk of pregnancy. Contraceptive methods can be made into scapegoats for loss of interest in sex.

Attitudes to the vaginal examination

Some women, particularly those belonging to the lower socio-economic groups and Irish Catholic women, have an aversion to 'the internal' which may prevent them getting contraceptive advice or finding fault with those methods which require it. They may allow a vaginal examination when pregnant but not at any other time. A woman is often afraid of what it may reveal about herself — it can reveal vulnerability and perhaps what she wishes to keep hidden even from herself, her own sexy feelings. She may be afraid that she will become excited during the examination. She has never been given permission nor given herself permission to explore her own body and feels guilty doing so. It is perhaps inevitable that women should have fantasies about this inner space — its size, texture, where it leads to, etc. — and it is therefore no accident that certain feminists have set up self-examination groups. By getting a woman to examine herself the doctor can give her permission to accept this part of herself as good.

Summing up

People who are secure in their identity, who do not need to prove femininity (or masculinity), who accept their genitals and sexual function as normal and healthy and who form trusting, warm, caring relationships and do not envy or resent or need to punish the opposite sex, and who value children as unique persons rather than cuddly dollies, may be concerned about the side-effects or drawbacks to the contraceptive methods but will settle on one and use it reliably. Problems with contraception, either in settling on a method or using it reliably or going from one method to another with complaints about each, will be seen in the person who lacks self-esteem, who is uncertain of their femininity or masculinity and needs the proof of children for reassurance, who is disgusted by the genitals and sexual function or who has a sexual difficulty, who cannot form intimate, trusting relationships and who envies or resents the opposite sex and who sees children as a means to an end. Individuals who are afraid of responsibility or have not developed inner control and resent outside authority may 'rebel' by finding contraception too much bother. Crises in the personal life or in the relationship can set up conflicts that lead to complaints about, or erratic use of, contraception. Thus, by complaining of problems with contraception, the person is often wanting to draw attention to other problems, e.g. in the relationship or with sex itself, which cannot be complained of directly or which the person may not be fully aware of or admit consciously. For the doctor to attempt to control the situation by forcing the person to make a choice without exploring deeper is to ignore a powerful cry for help.

25

Emotional significance of anxieties about the pill

Margaret Blair

Since 1973 I have seen between 4000 and 5000 patients requesting termination of pregnancy at Charing Cross Hospital. Almost all of them know about birth control and the majority have tried the pill at some time but have given it up or taken it irregularly. Some of the overt reasons given for this are realistic but many are a signal of other difficulties and anxieties.

It is therefore worthwhile, when a patient wants to give up the pill or is obviously projecting her fears on to it, to look a little closer into her circumstances. The verbalised anxieties until proven otherwise should lead the doctor to expect that the patient is having emotional problems either herself, or in the relationship with her partner.

Problems related to the patient herself

The need to prove or disprove her fertility. Patients who are not very certain in their own femininity and feel their sexuality might be damaging may project their fears of damage on to the pill, expressed as the damage they think the pill may do to them.

Clues that suggest this is the case may be other signs of uncertain femininity such as difficulty with menstruation, pregnancy or labour, or psychosexual difficulties.

Some of these patients really feel a need to test out their femininity by becoming pregnant.

Adolescent and immaturity problems. Many adolescents are reliable pill-takers but it is so often the ones who are having difficulties in other areas of their lives who declare that they can't take the pill — they get nausea, or gain weight. In the background there are often disturbed or broken homes, alcoholism and neglect or, by contrast, an overstrict attitude on the part of the parent. Both lead to a battle with the parents or authority figures, including the doctor, and the wish to demonstrate their developing sexuality and independence. Their need is to do this in an irresponsible way.

170

A way of asking for help. Not all patients can ask directly for help and understanding and may not even know what they are trying to get help for. They just know that they are under some sort of stress and are feeling increasingly resentful about having to take a pill every day. Many of these patients are expressing dependency problems.

Difficulty in the relationship with the partner
Anxieties projected onto the pill are very frequently a sign of stress in the relationship with the partner. When this stress is about the sexual side of the relationship it can be a cover for an actual dislike of intercourse and a wish to avoid it, or for frigidity. It can also be an expression of real problems such as impotence or premature ejaculation.

Probably difficulty in the relationship with the partner is the commonest cause of the projection of anxieties on to the pill. Many patients attending the termination clinic have given up the pill at the time that they need it most — that is when the relationship is on the point of breaking up. It should therefore be a warning to us all, when a patient is obviously projecting her fears onto the pill, to look more closely into her circumstances. Intervention at this stage, rather than collusion with the request, may prevent an unwanted pregnancy.

26
Youth advisory work

'What can you say to young people today?'

Fay Hutchinson

My first response to the question 'What can you say to young people today?' was 'What an arrogant title for a talk'. It seemed to imply that there is a magic formula or technique that allows you to communicate with the young — and by 'young' I mean under 18 year olds — and probably tell them what *you* think they ought to be doing. In observing myself at work, I realise that I don't actually talk to them very much; most of my effort is directed to trying to get *them* to talk, about themselves, why they've come to see me, what they want to do, what's causing them concern and what they can do to cope with it. Though I may not be talking much I am busy observing the patients, trying to assess them, responding to their needs, asking appropriate open-ended questions and giving them time to try and express themselves.

I would like to try and give you my particular viewpoint of some clinical encounters. Perhaps first, I should say something about my working conditions. I am a medical officer in the London Brook Advisory Centres, which have been developed to see young people who want contraception, or pregnancy counselling, or who are having problems in their sexual relationships, or with their family. Most of our work is in response to the request for birth control, but as we are well aware, this implies that an active sexual relationship is being anticipated, or followed, and provides an opening for discussion of sexual matters.

I think I am in a privileged position because most of our patients have *chosen* to come and see us, rather than their family doctor, and have an expectation that we are the right people to help them. Because of this, those who come are probably prepared to be more open with us than with someone who has a 'statutory' duty to them like their GP or a teacher or social worker. Indeed the relationship can be completely different with patients who are *brought* for us to do something to them, by a parent, or teacher or social worker who acts as the spokesman.

Case Study

Linda

For instance, I recall Linda, who was *brought* by her social worker when she was 14. Her parents

172

had split up some years before and when her mother became ill, Linda had to go into care. She was sullen, waif-like child who twisted about in the chair, wouldn't look at me, and looked bored while her social worker did the talking. The staff were worried because she seemed to be getting very involved with a 15-year-old boy in the home. He had been found in her bed, and I was asked to do a pregnancy test, examine her, and put her on the pill. Linda looked as though this had northing to do with her, and scowled. I realised I was not going to find out anything about her while there was someone talking for her, and I asked if I might see her on her own. After some reluctance — 'I don't think that's necessary' — I was left with Linda. I said she hadn't looked very happy with someone else talking about her, and asked if she would like to tell me what had happened, and how she felt I could help her. After a few sighs and squirms she began to talk, in a very small voice, not looking at me. She didn't like being in care and couldn't wait for mother to get better. She said the boy who had been found with her was a nuisance; he seemed to be after her all the time and she didn't even like him. He had threatened her when he came into her room and had 'tried to get his thing up her' but she had kept him away and had tried to call out, which is when the staff came in. She was angry and said there had been such a fuss she had given up trying to explain what had happened. She didn't have any intention of having sex with him and felt she was being made to go on the pill so that 'they wouldn't have to worry about her'. It took a while to get her to appreciate that she didn't have to do anything she didn't want to, that she should be able to tell the care staff if she was being pestered, and that I would only put her on the pill if she felt she needed it. It also took some time to persuade her social worker that Linda wanted support and would ask for contraception when she felt she needed it. During this session Linda had changed from being a sullen withdrawn child to an angry and frightened one who felt she couldn't control anything.

When she left she looked happier and bigger, more confident. She did come to see me two years later. She was still in the home, but had fallen in love with a boy at school. They were petting, and she decided to come and see me and go on the pill, because she was sure she was going to start sleeping with him. She wanted to, but didn't want to become pregnant. She had felt that because I had let her make her own decision before, she could come and talk to me again when she needed to.

The young present in infinite variety, but what of the doctor they meet? With this doctor they see a large, fat, aged woman with glasses, who probably looks as though she wouldn't have any idea of what they're talking about and is well past it. But during a clinical session this seems to be lost sight of. I suppose newcomers get some preparation because I go into the waiting room to fetch the next patient. I usually ask for them by their first name and I seem to be referred to as Fay, sometimes Dr Fay. Sometimes three girls get up when I call Karen or Susan, and perhaps the reaction from old friends who look quite happy to come in helps to make them feel it can't be so bad. Because they have come with a specific request it is easier to start talking. I may say 'Hello — what can I do for you?' This can throw them, they may not be used to asking for themselves, or expressing themselves but remarks like 'It's not very easy to put things into words', or 'How do *you* feel about it?' may help them to start. Each patient presents a new challenge. I am trying to assess from their manner and appearance what kind of a person they are. Are they happy and confident in what they're doing, or well defended from showing any feelings or anxiety? Sometimes the appearance is a shock — it's meant to be! Some of the young people can stir up feelings of hostility with their shaven heads and bizarre clothes.

There were two in the waiting room last week. They seemed to be standing around, menacing, in their leather jackets and Doc Martin boots, puffing away at their cigarettes. When the first came in I didn't recognise her, she was acting so tough. We had been seeing her for a year, since she had an abortion at 15. She had started truanting from school when her parents were breaking up, had now dropped out of school and was facing unemployment without any qualification with an 'aggressive resignation'. Once I had recognised her, I felt less disturbed by her, and she talked about her headaches on the pill, how she was bored and fed up about her parents. She had moved into a flat with her mate. Later, I did suggest she went to our counsellor, who would be able to see her more frequently, to see if we could find any way of helping her to put herself less at risk. She had really come that day to bring another mate, Dawn, to see us, because Dawn was scared to come on her own. Dawn was also 16, small inside her sheep-skin coat, with chrome yellow hair shaven on top, and a pin through her nose. She looked fearsome. Strangely, she made me feel motherly towards her, when I saw she was shaking. She had had an abortion at 14 after she had been raped, had been brought up by her mother, who didn't have much time for her, and mother was now moving in with a new boy friend who had children, and there wasn't room for Dawn. She had been kept on the pill by the frequent visits of the domiciliary family planning staff, had had a number of unfeeling sexual relationships but now had a boy friend she cared for. In the recent upheaval of leaving home she had lost her pills for three days, and her period hadn't come. When she undressed for examination, you could see the frightened little girl she was, who needed mothering and tenderness.

Studying the doctor-patient relationship I realise that 'mothering' is not the only role I have, though it is one I feel comfortable with, and many of the deprived youngsters I see may have need of this, especially if they are like Lana.

Case Study

Lana

Lana was the first illegitimate child of parents who did not accept her. She had been in care and fostered till she was 13, then rejoined her mother and extended family but never felt accepted. She had taken up with the 'motor-bike grease' and now had leather jacket and tattoos. Pregnant at 15, she was turned out of the home. She was determined to have her baby and bring her up herself. I have been seeing her for six years through a variety of crises. Inarticulate and a loser, she needed to feel she could always get in touch and share her misery. Against the odds, she was loving her little girl and stuck with her, determined not to let *her* lose her mother. Lucy is growing up a remarkably happy child with a devoted mother and I feel like her grandmother. Lana was sad that she could not understand why her mother could not show affection to her or Lucy. We talked about this.

The doctor-patient relationship

Sometimes the doctor-patient relationship is friendly and equal. Many of the young women I see are confident in their sexual relationships and enjoy their lives. They come for a good relationship with a 'mother' who can accept their feelings and sexuality.

Sometimes I can feel really put down by a patient. I had a very prim young woman who disapproved of sex before marriage, and would, I believed, feel the same after marriage. To her rage she had become pregnant as a result of heavy petting and intra-crural ejaculation. Her fiance and I were both made to feel dirty and humiliated in trying to find what she wanted to do about it, and were punished for our implied expectation that sexual intimacy was not unexpected in an engaged couple by her disdain and anger.

174

I sometimes feel despair and hopelessness when I learn of the horror and violence some of my patients experience. To a 16 year old: 'You look upset today' — 'Yes, my fella's up for armed robbery'. To a giggly 14 year old: 'How did you get your black eye?' — 'I was attacked and when my friend tried to get him off me, he drew a knife and got her in the arm; we're going to court today'.

Commenting on appearance or behaviour can often provide an opportunity to discuss fears and anxieties that might otherwise not be expressed. A silent, hostile girl was noticably uncommunicative about how she became pregnant, and about her boy friend. When I said 'You look very unhappy, and I can see you don't want to talk about this', she burst out with 'Of course I don't, it's my father'.

We may gain insight about the patients' feelings, about their sexuality, from the response to a genital examination. In young patients who come for contraception and have no symptoms, I do not feel obliged to insist on a vaginal examination before prescribing, but the response to the question, 'Would you like me to examine you?', will show if they can accept and use the vagina, or have fears or anxieties about it. These may be discussed, especially a fear of pain or being too small, and sometimes examination can be offered to observe their reaction and sometimes explore their fears and fantasies. Most girls are pleased to learn that they are fine and healthy, but to insist on examination can be humiliating and painful experience to someone who still feels her genitals are very private and is only just learning to use and share them.

In our multicultural society we meet people with beliefs and expectations quite different from our own. Communication may be even more difficult if there is a language barrier, but the difficulties caused by cultural differences need attention. I am seeing more girls from a strictly controlled upbringing, Hindu, Moslem or Roman Catholic, who are rebelling against their parents' beliefs and trying to be like their contemporaries. Because of their lack of preparation, and parental rejection if they are discovered, they are at great risk and need great care, and because of the taboo on premarital sexual intercourse they have great difficulty recognising their own need for contraception.

Many of the young black people are very wary and reserved when they first attend. They seem to wear a mask, are 'respectful' but don't look at you. If they feel welcome and at home they can begin to allow their own personality to show, and may seem different people when they come next time.

I haven't said anything yet about the young men we see, and that could be a separate talk. On the whole the sexual welfare of boys is neglected. They don't have the same access as girls to professional advice for contraception, or pregnancy. We see a number who come as partners and use this as an opportunity to discuss sexual matters.

They may be supportive and considerate, or they may be excluded and made to feel useless. Since we have encouraged young men to come to the centres on their own to get contraceptives, and treat them responsibly as we do the girls, they are being seen by the counsellors and medical staff. To begin with they like to come as a gang, rather as the younger girls do: they feel safer with their mates for support, and can treat it all as a bit of a joke. I sometimes feel that coming to Brook is becoming part of a South London initiation rite, and the reception staff have had to think out the way they welcome and cope with five or fifteen young men who crash in and ask if they can join, and can they have some Durex? They are individually registered as patients, and asked to see the counsellor, who is one of our specially trained social workers. About 50 per cent will agree to be seen, and these are mostly those who are having or hoping to have a sexual relationship. When they are seen, individually or with their friends, and given an opportunity to talk for themselves, they are able to reveal anxieties about themselves, their performance or their relationships, and will use the chance to discuss them. One of the commonest fears is not being 'big enough' to satisfy the girl, or of being laughed at because the penis is 'too small'. Sometimes they can be helped by discussion to understand that the value of an erect penis is what use is made of it, rather than bemoaning the size of the flaccid penis. Occasionally we are asked to examine the genitals — I feel, to pass them fit for service, because of fears about their normality. The young man may be extremely tense and anxious, and so may the doctor, but as with the genital examination of women, when the clothes are removed, this may be the time when fears and fantasies can be expressed — about the size (always 'too small'), damage from circumcision, or a tight foreskin, deviation from the mid-line, one testicle being lower than the other, or bigger or absent. Usually, listening to the fears expressed and accepting the normality of the genitals is therapeutic.

Counselling boys
We have heard a great deal about women's lack of sexual satisfaction in the last few years, and some of our young men feel incapable from the start, because if they can't 'make her come' right away, they can't be any good as a sexual partner, and the fear is that girls will talk and *everyone* will know they're no good. Instant sexual success is thought to be the goal and the obvious relief that comes during discussion of the need to learn and discover from each other appears to increase confidence.

During adolescence there is a great need to be accepted, to be normal if not supernormal compared to your peers, and anyone who falls outside the prevailing norm can become depressed and withdrawn. Despite the efforts that have been made to make homosexuality more widely understood and accepted, young people who find that their sexual interests are predominantly homosexual can feel isolated and hopeless if they cannot accept this in themselves, or see any way of living a tolerable life as a homosexual.

I remember a case that presented dramatically at a very busy Youth Advisory Centre one evening. There was a commotion outside. Irate parents had brought in their self-satisfied 14-year-old daughter who had been disturbed with a 15-year-old boy. They were wanting to involve the police and get immediate pregnancy tests. I was struck by her complacency and smugness, and suggested I saw her on her own. She was scornful and said of course nothing had happened; he couldn't make it. I later saw the boy on his own. He was a big, fresh-cheeked, good-looking 15 year old, near to tears, who slowly began to talk after I had asked him gently if he would like to tell me what had happened. The situation had been set up by some of his mates who were sure he was 'queer' because he didn't want to go with girls, and with the connivance of the 14 year old, who was well known as being available. He was being given his chance to prove himself, and now not only had he failed, but he would be known to have failed publicly. He felt he couldn't face school again, and life wouldn't be worth living if he was gay. The immediate crisis of the girl and her parents was sorted out, but David needed immediate support in his desperation. I felt he could well make a suicide attempt — this is not uncommon in young homosexuals — and was able to contact a sympathetic youth worker used to working with young homosexuals who was able to see him more frequently while he came to terms with himself.

Conclusion

I realise I have said little specifically about 'psychosexual problems'. On the whole, young people do not present themselves with a 'sexual problem'. They are more likely to be worried about their desirability as a sexual partner, whether their bodies are normal and attractive. They may be anxious about their performance and ability to 'satisfy', but if there is a failure, it is usually attributed to the relationship and they seek a new partner. Much of their anxiety at this age is in accepting their own sexual desires and performance and separating from their parents. Sexual problems as such are not usually recognised until they reach their twenties.

I have no formula for talking to young people. If there was one I think I would be very bored with the work. Each clinical encounter is a challenge that may require all our skills if we are going to take full advantage of it.

27

Seminars and youth advisory work

Gillian Hinshelwood

I work in Camden, which is rightly proud of its caring facilities for all groups of citizens, and young people are no exception. There are good GPs, hospitals, youth clubs, schools, Social Services, and many more informal help organisations. All these are well publicised and well used.

It is the knowledge of the existence of such facilities that allows me to feel comfortable in stepping back to look beyond the requests presented in our clinics, and to ask: Why this patient, at this time, here, with this particular problem?

Case Study

Miss A.

> Miss A. presented to discuss birth control. She had been referred, and was accompanied by another patient of mine whom I had known for eight years — a confident young woman. Miss A. was shy and rather respectful. She considered the methods of birth control intelligently and chose to be fitted with a cap, which was no trouble. The disconcerting thing in all this was that Miss A. was aged 41, and came from Wiltshire especially for the appointment. She had many quite acceptable reasons for doing this. However, in spite of them all, and almost because of the way she justified herself, it seemed worth remarking that I felt as if I were being asked to treat her as a youthful person, uncertain of her sexual development. She livened up at this, and talked with considerable emotion about her sheltered childhood, her caring for her widowed invalid mother until her death nine months ago, keeping her affair with a divorced German a secret, wishing for a fling and still fearful of venturing forth.

Our patients present us with an enormous and formidable range of requests and problems, but it seems to me that if they come to a centre that implies by its name that it concerns itself with *youth* they are stating that they wish to get help, or to discuss some aspect of their involvement in the tasks of adolescence, and I think all the patients we see can be considered in this way. The tasks of adolescence are:

1. To reach an appropriate level of education, and decide on a career.
2. To separate from parental dependence.
3. To relate to a peer group.
4. To reach physical maturity and be fairly satisfied with the result.
5. To form a mature sexual identity and make a satisfying heterosexual relationship.

I think that what the seminars best equip me for is to identify first, then help, those young people who are confused by and cannot cope with these tasks. This is done by giving them an experience of being listened to without any guidance or direction. The experience of stopping and looking, whether one is going uphill or downhill, is frightening at any age, but never worse than in adolescence when there is such internal and external pressure for movement. Left to their own devices, most young people will act rather than reflect, but will request practical help. There are countless instances where practical intervention is appropriate, but the priority is listening, in an attempt to understand, using the doctor-patient relationship and the material offered. This gives the person the safety to dare to risk looking at his distress and confusion, rather than avoiding them. It is also very pleasant to be able to recognise that in some cases no serious conflict is present, and to enjoy a friendly contact or referral. Because of this, I feel strongly that the initial contact in such an agency should, if possible, be with the most experienced workers, rather than the other way round.

Case Study

Mr B. and Miss C.

Mr B. and Miss C. were referred by a GP and I was the fifth person they had seen. They met on an overland trip from Australia, and their troubles began in Europe. For the same presenting symptoms, on different occasions, he was treated for gastro-intestinal upset, respiratory infection and depression, and she for an anxiety state. They were referred to me for treatment of their sex problem. Miss C. did nearly all the talking at first, and poured out her fears of not being sexy enough, wondering if she was making him impotent, talking at length about the good and bad aspects of their relationship. He was much quieter, and concerned himself with trying to reassure her that he was fond of her and that he was sure that sex was not the problem. When asked about himself, he just said that for the last two weeks he had been feeling more and more ill and indeed he looked most unwell. He had no energy for anything, and every two days he had a bad fever which left him shivering and miserable. He did not think he was impotent, just ill. I referred him to the Hospital for Tropical Diseases where he was admitted immediately with malaria. This was treated, and he was fine afterwards. Miss C. continued to see me for a few weeks while they were in England as she did have the problem of her lack of confidence in her femininity.

Relief of anxiety and distress, and avoidance of further pain are the patient's priorities, and it is easy to make them one's own, seeing the youth as a vulnerable son or daughter. So we launch enthusiastically into teaching, treating, reassuring — all good defences, as we have learned in our seminars — and liaising. Once I get involved in liaising with other workers, I know that I have no real understanding of the patient any more than he or she has. I do not mean making a definite referral, such as to a VD clinic or to an accommodation agency, but the more ill-defined rumblings that can take place between various departments and organisations caring for young people. I think the much easier task of understanding and relating to the colleague is substituted for that of understanding the patient, who can get left out in the cold.

Case Study

Jane

Jane is 16½, is in care and has been for much of her life, and has lived in a succession of children's homes. She was referred for birth-control advice, which she agreed she wanted as she had a boy

179

friend. She keeps her appointments and has no trouble with the pill, is likeable and friendly and talks easily, but is non-committal about anything serious. On at least four occasions, however, her social worker has spent a lot of time on the phone asking me to help Jane with her sexuality, as they are worried by her behaviour. I feel on each occasion that I can understand the social worker perfectly, and resolve to try! Jane shows none of this problem to me, however hard I feel I try, and I think she is telling me that in this aspect of her life she is coping, and she is, if the way she conducts her session with me shows the least bit of her. I try to tell social workers that I can only work with what I am given, and encourage them to work with the aspect that worries them.

It is very easy to start identifying with other adults in the patient's life, and I find the seminar discipline most valuable in helping me resist the temptation of directing the patient's behaviour, supposedly to spare the parents' anguish.

Case Study

Sally

Sally was an untidy, boisterous looking girl of nearly 18 who was referred by her teacher. She had been a promising pupil, considered easily able to cope with the four A-levels that she needed to be a vet, but her performance had deteriorated over the last year, and she walked out of two exams. She talked readily, almost explosively, about her various thoughts, in a very disjointed way. Her sisters had rebelled, and she did not want to disappoint her parents. She wanted to train horses. She thought she would like to be an artist because she was obsessed with women's bodies. She had a holiday job in Sainsbury's and it was a new and exciting world. Her sister was married to a man who was paralysed down one side. She was a likeable and intelligent girl and it was difficult not to encourage her not to waste her talents, determined as she seemed to stay in Sainsbury's for ever. But she must have had many people around her voicing those sentiments, and I put this to her in those terms and she said yes, they all thought she was lazy, but she was so hard-worked inside. I have seen her fortnightly over the last two months, and she does seem disenchanted with shop work and much more settled in her plan to accept an art school foundation place.

The very strict discipline in seminars of only looking at the patient, doctor and presentation, never comparing, never referring to theory, achieves the best understanding of the situation and the best chances of a successful outcome with any patient. An adolescent is very engaged in creating an independent identity for himself, and can be particularly affronted, or feel misunderstood, if in our interviews we resort to generalisations. On the other hand, young people beg to be reassured that they are like all the others. All the more reason, therefore, to conduct the interview with careful concentration on the material given and the doctor-patient relationship, rather than make assumptions which may not be valid.

Finally, if I am really careful to stick to the discipline learned in the seminars. I find it helps me to avoid two major pitfalls in working with young people. One of these is allowing them to harbour and develop a grudge which can be made responsible for all the misfortunes of life, such as a wicked stepmother, or bat ears. The other pitfall is encouraging one or both of you to feel that salvation lies only in you, and the contribution of all the other people who have helped to shape the person's life is negligible. This can only lead to disappointment all round, and can be avoided by really listening to the material given and by using the doctor-patient relationship.

28

The use of seminar training in general practice

Peter Mitford

To an extent the use of seminar training in general practice is the same as its use in any other branch of medicine as we are all trying to achieve the same end using similar methods. It is the setting which is somewhat different in general practice, leading principally to a difference in style and emphasis. This paper will concern itself with an attempt to indicate how the seminar training has been modified for use in this setting.

Why seminar training is useful for general practitioners
First, the experience of a Balint group is invaluable in every field of medicine. This experience has dramatically altered my approach to the patient and my understanding of the nature of the consultation. Were I never to see another patient with sexual problems, I would still regard the experience as an invaluable one and probably the most useful piece of postgraduate training I have ever undertaken.

Second, the training has been of use to me as a clinical assistant in problem-orientated family planning counselling at the local general hospital. Anyone working in this field should be aware of the presentation of psychosexual problems which inevitably turn up in disguise in this setting.

Third, in general practice itself I was conscious of the need to do a little more than cough, shuffle and recommend gin for patients with sexual problems.

Problems during the training period
My main problem was to have sufficient cases 'on the go' to fill the needs of the seminar group. This sometimes meant the presentation of a case which was only half prepared and sometimes when I was still genuinely uncertain whether the problem was truly psychosexual.

The first contact with the patient was usually made in a normal surgery session either during the course of a consultation, or by referral from one of my partners. After spending sufficient time to establish a rapport and show the patient that I was concerned to help, he/she was brought back when there was sufficient time to go into the amount of detail required. I tended to continue to bring the patient back at such specially allocated times for follow-up when I could also see their spouses if this seemed appropriate.

Now all of this sounds all right, except that it makes no use of the special advantages which general practice has over all other branches of medicine. Later I evolved my own system of working in general practice, which for reasons I will outline, has distinct advantages.

Areas of particular therapeutic advantage in general practice

1. Patients seeing a general practitioner can remain both 'anonymous' and 'respectable'. Consider my situation in a small market town. An unmarried 16 year old requires family planning advice. There is an excellent family planning clinic in the town but if she sits in the waiting room she immediately broadcasts her purpose to the rather insular community. She may well find that she is sitting beside her mother or her married sister. On the other hand she may make an appointment to see me and sit in my waiting room with absolute confidence that there is no way in which anyone can foresee her reason for being there.

    If one expands the argument from family planning to psychosexual problems where the need for confidentiality is even greater, one can see the advantage of being able to consult one's own general practitioner.

    Some patients with sexual difficulties would prefer not to confide in their family doctor. There are many reasons: (a) Personal friendship. (b) Unapproachability. (c) Embarrassment. (d) The patient sees too much of him in other areas of his family care to wish to involve him in this area. (e) The patient may not think much of the doctor or may not consider that he could have any expertise in this field.

2. However, there are areas where the general practitioner's understanding of the family dynamic may be of particular help. Consider a situation of potential trouble of which I am aware. Joe is of Italian extraction and owns a small business close to the town. The business was inherited from father who established it and built it up during the very difficult time just after Second World War internment. Joe lives with father who is now retired and a very domineering stepmother who is the classical 'fat Italian Moma' and totally in charge at home.

    Father, to escape from the noise and aggravation, has retreated quietly into alcoholism. Joe escapes by working night and day. He has met and just married a nice but very shy good Catholic girl who has moved into the family home. There is already a problem as she does not want a child for a few years but wishes to use only methods of contraception approved by the Church. She has interpreted too literally the local priest's advice to 'follow her conscience' and see her doctor. No sexual problem has yet emerged, but should she begin to complain of vaginal discharge with no findings on examination or other anxiety symptoms, my ears will be very open to the cry for help beneath the surface.

GPs are uniquely placed to predict trouble and initiate early action which may prevent the trouble becoming a major one and therefore more difficult to deal with.

I now try to exploit this advantage by dealing with the problem as it presents in the same way as I deal with all other problems. The patient is seen during a routine surgery and brought back for review during other normal surgery hours, perhaps with a somewhat extended appointment. This, I think, helps the patient to view the problem as one requiring medical help like all others and not to regard him or herself as being extraordinary. My consultation is different from that in a clinic because I already have much background information. I am usually familiar with the patient's housing situation, the number in the family, relationships between them, the patient's employment and financial position, etc.

There is little difficulty with follow-up. It can be as frequent and as long as I consider necessary. But, if therapeutic efforts are of no avail, I do not hesitate to call a halt. This was a major problem for me in the early stages.

Results

As may be expected, the results by and large have improved with greater experience. The early cases I think often sensed my anxiety. They had special sessions set aside for them which reinforced their beliefs that they were freaks or that something was seriously wrong. I spent much time exploring blind alleys.

As time has gone by I have been able to get to the bones of the cases more speedily.

Even so my results have varied from the extremely successful to total failure. The outstandingly successful case I recall was of one session of 20 minutes with a couple presenting. The complaint was of recent onset of intermittent impotence. The husband was in his late forties and his wife in her early forties. Both had been married before. There was an extremely good relationship between them and they communicated easily. Since intermittent impotence had started, tension had been building up in the wife. Her previous husband had been a sexual athlete. It proved very easy to defuse the situation with discussion and some simple advice. There was a grateful phone call later saying that all was well and that follow-up was unnecessary. One wonders if the result would have been as satisfactory if the couple had had to wait for counselling in a special clinic.

There was a moderately good result with a male patient in his late fifties. His first marriage had broken up whilst he was in his early twenties. Since that time his sexual experience had been limited to masturbation and casual sex. He had now retired and met a widow in her late forties. They both wished to marry but he had proved to be impotent. He was obviously under considerable pressure to succeed as this was the first meaningful relationship he had had in a very long time. In this case a combination of counselling with sensate focusing on the Masters & Johnson principle led to an improvement. Thereafter he had some difficulty with premature ejaculation which again was helped by the squeeze technique. After some little time they were having a regular and relatively satisfactory sexual relationship. He made an interesting comment on the use of sensate focusing and other Masters &

Johnson type techniques. 'It is all very well in the centrally heated hotels in the States doctor, but you should try all this business in Northumberland in January in a back bedroom with a small electric fire!' One had visions of a most unusual case of frostbite.

At the other end of the scale though, there was a most unsuccessful session with a crushed impotent little man who was frog-marched into the surgery by his large domineering wife to 'get fixed'. She frightened the life out of me too. During discussion it was apparent that there was no worthwhile relationship between them. She left quite disgusted that he did not get potency pills and they did not come back for review.

There were also some inappropriate cases where the psychosexual difficulties proved to have arisen because of marital difficulties instead of the other way round. These I found extremely difficult to sort out in the early days. They have not done very well by and large and in several cases the marriage has broken up.

I have had three cases whose presenting symptom was impotence and who were subsequently found to have an organic disease. One is dead, having had a bronchogenic carcinoma. One is handicapped by partial blindness and peripheral neuritis due to diabetes. One has gout and has had deep-vein thromboses. He is suspected of having occult malignancy. He has been carefully investigated but as yet no underlying mitotic lesion has been found.

29

Vasectomy counselling

S. A. Corrin

The setting in which I see patients is a community health clinic for vasectomy counselling in South London set in the midst of a large number of council estates.

Couples are always seen and a medical history of both taken. During the interview the direct question is asked 'Have you any sexual problems?' but sexual problems can be picked up or suspected at various other points in the interview.

The first problem noted may be the alarm when the husband sees that a woman doctor is doing the counselling. The shyness between male patient and woman doctor in this situation may sometimes reflect shyness and lack of communication between husband and wife in their marital and sexual life.

Sexual problems may be recognised when I ask about the contraceptive history and reason for wanting vasectomy. Perhaps a wife says, somewhat angrily, 'Well, I've taken all the trouble up to now and had to do everything. It's his turn now. He's the one who always wants it' (i.e. sex). Or from the husband, 'We don't want any more children. The wife's always tired. There's so much work to do with the children: up at night. She's worn out. You can't expect her to be interested in sex, so we want vasectomy.'

In the medical and obstetric history sexual problems are again recognised, e.g. the quite common mention of postnatal depression, for which professional advice has not always been sought in spite of being noted, and an accompanying loss of libido.

In a recent case the history plus presentation gave a graphic picture of psychosexual problems: a woman of 26 with two children, one miscarriage and one termination of pregnancy in her first marriage, coming with her second husband, aged 23, and the six-month-old child of this marriage, wanting vasectomy. She didn't like any methods of contraception she had had and she had tried them all and changed them frequently. Her husband would use sheaths but she didn't like them; vasectomy was the method for her. Questioned about whether she had considered sterilisation for herself, she said she would not consider it; she's been through enough.

One may detect problems in the way couples reply to a direct question about psychosexual problems. A confident united reply of 'No, no problems at all' with a big smile at each other is very convincing. But other couple's replies are less convincing and one may suspect but not always pick up the problem, 'I don't think we've a problem, have we?' from the husband looking at the wife, and then she replies 'No, I don't think so'; or 'No, I don't think so really', said rather slowly.

One husband said to his wife 'Have we any problems dear?'; there was a pause, then he said 'Have we any do you think?' and after a long pause she slowly and obviously reluctantly said 'Well, yes, I'm not very interested in sex'.

One husband said 'No, no we've no problems'. But, as the wife was silent, I asked her again and she burst into tears to the astonishment of her husband and admitted to loss of any pleasure in sex since the onset of her first and only pregnancy two years before. She was 35 and it was her first marriage but her husband's second. She had hidden it and the depression from him for two years. She had previously had a 'wonderful' sex life with him for several years.

When psychosexual problems are discovered at vasectomy counselling, opportunities to get help with them are always offered, but I find they are very rarely taken up. Presumably this is because the patients are not complaining of them. They have been discovered by the doctor. The patients have accepted them and incorporated them into their lives, without too much pain.

Here is a case that did come for help.

Case Study

Mr and Mrs L., aged 47 and 45, came to the clinic to talk about vasectomy. He was a sound-recording engineer, a tall, burly man, ruddy-complexioned and formally dressed for the interview. She was short, slight and pale with dark hair. She had been attending the family planning clinic for some years and was taking the pill. The wife started talking but soon her husband took over. He wanted his wife to come off the pill and he wanted to have a vasectomy. Mrs L. said she had no problems with the pill and I had a strong feeling that Mr L. wasn't really concerned about his wife's health, but had come to get vasectomy done for himself. Then he said 'But I've heard it's not a good idea to have vasectomy done if there are problems'. He couldn't get an erection now. The problem had started suddenly about two years before. His GP had sent him for tests on faeces, urine and blood but they had found nothing wrong with him. His GP had given him some vitamin tablets but there had been no improvement.

At first, he said, he had a few spontaneous erections which did not last long enough for successful intercourse, but that masturbation by his wife or himself did not bring on an erection even when continued 'for a long time'. He couldn't 'get any sensation in his penis'.

He had no business or financial worries now or in the past and had had the same job for years.

I agreed that vasectomy was not advisable until this problem had been sorted out and suggested another appointment.

I was very worried about whether I shouldn't have sent him straight away for more physical investigations, because of the possibility that this might not be a psychosexual problem. I think some of the anxiety in me was a result of the impression that he was the sort of man who did not believe in psychological problems. They were a sign of weakness and he gave the outward impression of being a powerful dominating man.

An appointment was arranged to fit in with one of his trips abroad but not kept and not cancelled.

Some months later they phoned for another appointment to see me with no mention of the previous appointment. I was surprised when only Mr L. came into the room. I asked about his wife and he said she was outside, but he wanted to see me on his own first. He straight away began to talk quite uninhibitedly about his problem and went on for a long time.

He had had 'no pleasure' from sex for about two years. Up till then he had led an active sex life, having intercourse about four times a week. While he travelled abroad he had 'sex all the time'. His trouble began suddenly. He had difficulty getting erections and his penis felt numb. He had occasionally woken in the night with an erection and tried straight away to have intercourse but the erection soon failed, and eventually he got none at all, even after masturbating.

By contrast, he used to get erections very easily at any time, e.g. 'at the sight of a girl across the street'. I felt that he had been very proud of his sexual prowess and felt he was 'sexier' than most men of his age. He told me what he had done to try and help himself; pornography in books and films, sex shops and sex clubs in Denmark, sex with different women in various settings (including groups), but nothing had made any difference.

Though I had some admiration for his energy and drive (though it also probably showed how desperate he felt), these descriptions made me feel inadequate and ignorant and rather prim. I hoped he would not ask me any questions and expose my ignorance of some of the things he was talking about. I was also acutely aware of the contrast between the places he had been to and the one we were in — a clinic in a converted council flat, slightly the worse for wear, as I felt I myself looked late in the evening, sitting in front of a wall covered with large pink and blue kittens chasing balls of knitting wool across the wallpaper (the clinic is also a children's clinic). I felt he'd been to all the more likely places for help on his list first and was down to his last hope. After all he'd done, what could the doctor do now?

When he stopped talking I asked him questions because I didn't know what to do next.

He'd been married for 25 years and had three children, including a daughter of 19 with whom he didn't get on. She was a moody girl and did not approve of him. There had been a lot a family quarrels while she had been at home. I wondered if this could be related to his problem, because of the timing.

His father was dead. He had left Mr L.'s mother at 58 and gone off with another woman. Mr L. said his father was a 'gay man' and that he took after him. His mother lived near him but this was accidental he said.

He described his relationship with his wife as 'very close'. They were taken for 'brother and sister'. This seems an odd remark but I did not question it then. He said she enjoyed sex and they had no inhibitions about it, though he said in some ways she was not as good sexually as some of the women he had been with. I noticed myself feeling angry with him then at what I felt was a disparaging remark about his wife.

I tried to discover any physical basis for the impotence and he spontaneously said that his 'penis and balls had always been small' but that 'erection makes it normal'. I remember feeling pleased to recognise this first overt sign of anxiety; I had something to work with. I realised that physical examination would be important, but I felt anxious about doing it.

I asked him what made him think they were small and he started talking about sizes of penis, erect and non-erect, including the size of the largest erect penis he had heard of, the dimensions of which sounded incredible. I made no comment at all about this but thought that his need for such knowledge might be a sign of anxiety about his adequacy as a male.

I went on to check another possible source of anxiety and asked if he had ever wondered if the impotence had something to do with his age. He replied that he had 'wondered about this'. I said that increasing age never affected sex in this way and sexual intercourse continued normally into old age with no sudden stop.

I asked to examine him and he undressed and lay on the couch. I felt extremely apprehensive. I found no abnormality on examination and told him so.

I'd become aware of the lack of emotional feelings in him. It seemed as though this lack of feeling in life generally had now spread into his sexual life. We talked about it.

There was a noise outside. He was very alarmed and said 'Is that my wife? Could she have overheard what we've been saying? She doesn't know anything about what I've told you'. (It was hard to believe that a wife with this kind of husband wouldn't be suspicious of his extramarital activities.) I felt the need to reassure him that she wouldn't have been able to hear anything though I could not be sure about this as she was the last patient in the clinic.

I asked him to bring her in for a short talk before making another appointment to see them, but he came back on his own and said she did not want to come in as it was now so late. I asked if she was upset because she hadn't been called in earlier and he said 'No', but she was tired and she'd like to come and see me at the next appointment.

He came in for the next appointment two weeks later looking more carefully groomed than before and quite cool and collected. His wife was not with him. Mr L. said she didn't feel there was any point in her coming. I asked if she was upset because she hadn't been seen at the last appointment and he said 'Not at all'. I asked him how he was and how was the sexual problem. He said 'It's all right now. We've had sex normally four or five times. Sensation wasn't absolutely as perfect as it used to be but was almost so once or twice'. I was extremely surprised to hear this, and said I was pleased. He said it very 'matter-of-factly'. He went on to say that he didn't understand how such an improvement could have happened after one interview with me and said 'I am a bit of a male chauvinistic pig', which I later felt was as near as he could get to an acknowledgment that the doctor might have been helpful to him.

I suggested we tried to understand how this change had come about and we talked about how well hidden his anxiety had been from the doctor and probably from himself, and how little emotion he showed. I wasn't hopeful about the continuance of the potency and suggested another appointment, but he couldn't see any point in it, and he was going abroad shortly. He asked about the possibility of vasectomy being done before this and I said it could not be arranged in the time. Professionally I felt he should wait longer in any case though I did not say so.

Six weeks later his wife asked for coil insertion and said they had decided on this method of contraception for the present. I said I was sorry I hadn't seen her previously and she said 'It doesn't seem to have mattered because we're perfectly all right now'. In follow-ups over 18 months normal sex is still reported by her.

I felt that the sudden improvement in potency meant that the problem had possibly been due to an incident causing anxiety and loss of confidence in his sexuality, which had now been relieved; and that the opportunity to talk freely about the problem, and to feel that it had been respected, had restored his confidence. Possibly it was also important that a female doctor had been involved.

I could appreciate also the way he had managed to help himself by using the vasectomy interview to present his problem, and his ability to keep me absolutely silent during large parts of the interview.

188

30

Requests for abortion

Ruth E. Coles

Many aspects of counselling women who are seeking an abortion are the same as psychosexual counselling. One must watch and listen, not only to the words, but to what is really being said. But some aspects are different.

The first and most important difference is the time factor. All abortion counselling is urgent and must be completed in a few days; if you are lucky you may have a couple of weeks. You are constantly aware that if termination is to be carried out it must be done as early as possible. There is now evidence that if the cervix is dilated before ten weeks the risk of cervical incompetence is negligible, but it is likely to be even less at eight weeks and before this no dilation at all will be necessary. With this in mind, it is sometimes helpful to arrange termination first and then proceed with the counselling. This has two effects: no time is lost if a decision for termination is made, and the patient is more likely to be relaxed and to talk more freely without anxiety about making a good case in order to get what she thinks she wants. If, after counselling, a decision is made to continue the pregnancy then appointments are easily cancelled or transferred to someone else. The pressure of the time factor is particularly great when a patient presents at 10–12 weeks when any delay in the decision may mean the difference between a vaginal and a prostaglandin termination.

The second difference is that there is a decision to be made. In psychosexual counselling the aim is a change in attitude or an improvement in performance; there is no decision to be made except to seek and accept help and at any time the patient can opt out and decide that she would rather live with the problem than accept therapy. But for the woman with an unplanned pregnancy any opting out means that the pregnancy continues, and that is not a problem that can be hidden or ignored; it will grow and be obvious to all. There is no opting out for the doctor either. I am aware, when I am seeing psychosexual patients, that the counselling I do is better on some days than on others. Providing you have not been so useless that the patient has gone away in disgust, you will get another chance. Time factors do not allow for second chances in pregnancy counselling and wrong decisions may be made and implemented. If a patient comes back depressed and full of regrets about her termination, you have failed and all you can offer is support while she works through her grief. Both the time factor and the need for a definite decision put great pressure on the patient and the doctor.

There are other outside pressures. In psychosexual counselling not many people are involved. Pregnancy is often a more public affair which involves not only the partner but also parents, relatives, friends, colleagues, teachers, neighbours and even bosses, and they all feel the need to give good advice, most often: 'This was unintended, get rid of it, start again and pretend nothing has happened.' Reaching the patient's real feelings when she is being bombarded by so much 'common sense' is often difficult. The patient knows that her pregnancy will only remain a secret if it is ended and this is another sort of pressure. Many pregnancies are ended to hide the fact from parents and sometimes from partners too. Mothers who have 'nerves' are a problem, as are fathers who have had a coronary thrombosis; they must not be upset.

Case Study

I recently had a patient who came when she was nine weeks pregnant. She had been with her partner for four years. He was a married man and her boss. Later he became divorced and, thinking they would get married, my patient tried to get pregnant. Then the relationship began to deteriorate; they felt this was because of the difficulties of their boss-employee situation and the girl left her job. The relationship did not improve but they continued to see each other occasionally and in these unhappy circumstances pregnancy occurred. The girl instinctively felt that she wanted her baby but was uncertain whether marriage would be offered or if it would be suitable if it was. She hadn't told her partner about the pregnancy and I suggested that she should, so that she could find out what his reaction was instead of guessing at it. But the biggest obstacle to continuing the pregnancy was mother who had had several nervous breakdowns and might well have another in response to her daughter's extramarital pregnancy. I said that many mothers became happy grandmothers in spite of the particular circumstances. It seemed likely that mother would find some way of having her next breakdown, and as she was likely to live for another 20–30 years I asked my patient if she was prepared to make all her decisions concerning her adult life according to mother's nerves. The patient returned two days later to say that her partner was delighted about the pregnancy and they were considering marriage; mother didn't seem to matter any more.

Doctors are under other pressures too. Abortions are legal but no one has to do them. No one wants women to have unwanted children but no one wants to terminate pregnancies. We have enormous cooperation locally but I sometimes feel that I spend more time on the telephone making arrangements than I spend counselling the patient. The patient is the only person who matters but gynaecologists must be kept happy too.

A third difference between psychosexual and abortion counselling is the amount of information the patient needs. In psychosexual counselling patients have the basic information. Abortion is different. People have not thought about it because it is not likely to happen to them, or they have thought only on a very theoretical level and so one often hears 'I always thought it was wrong until now'. Attitudes change when an unwanted pregnancy has to be faced. Whatever the patient thinks about abortion she is unlikely to have much knowledge about the procedures and the risks and these must be explained.

As always, the way the patient presents is both interesting and significant. Our pregnancy advisory service is run alongside a contraceptive service and when it started ten years ago our staff were excellent at tactfully finding out whether requests for appointments were from girls needing contraception or girls already pregnant. They picked up the clues, and they nearly always got it right. Today it is acceptable to ask directly. Occasionally a patient seeking abortion turns up in a routine contraceptive session because she has been too frightened to explain, but this is unusual. Most patients are obviously women who know what they want and are coming to get it. Other appointments are made by parents or partners and the motivation of these patients is less obvious.

Most patients enter the consulting room alone, but some ask if they can bring their partner, parent or friend. Friends, or sometimes older sisters, are used for moral support and indicate that the patient feels unable to face you or her situation alone. Partners and parents may be used for moral support too, but the girl who brings her mother may be telling you that she is not mature enough to cope alone. This is hardly surprising if the girl is 14 or 15 but is more significant at 23 or 24. The presence of the partner may mean that this is a mature couple who feel that the decision about a pregnancy should be shared or it may be that the woman has insisted that he should accompany her because it is the least he can do and he must suffer too in a situation where he has left her 'holding the baby'. Which of these two roles are played is often evident from his manner. Sometimes the patient appears closely followed by an uninvited partner or parent with an air of determination which makes it clear that they are going to have their say, and you know whose feelings are going to be presented unless you handle the situation carefully.

Patients are self-selecting and the majority of those that seek our help at the Brook Clinic are asking for termination. A few are ambivalent and want help in making their decision and some come seeking permission to continue their pregnancies in the presence of opposition from those around them.

Some demand termination and hardly want to discuss it. They say I'm pregnant but I can't have it'. They will say no more about it without persuasion and you are made to feel an intruder as you try to reach their feelings. You rapidly find that 'can't have it' means 'don't want it'. Their decision is made and definite, maternity is totally unacceptable. Others say 'I'm pregnant and I can't have it because ...'; they go on to produce 101 practical reasons why the pregnancy cannot be continued, often red herrings. The practical difficulties of any unplanned pregnancy are obvious and easy for the patient to express. Reaching the feelings behind these practicalities and getting the patient to express them is more difficult. Sometimes it helps to ask her what her immediate reaction was to the confirmation of pregnancy. Some are able to let you know that they felt little pleasure before they were overtaken by the practical horrors; others tell you that the horrors started at once. Some give you a glimpse of their feelings in such expressions as 'Mum thinks it would be best', 'We can't get married yet', or 'My husband says we can't afford it'. This way of talking about the practicalities clearly tells you that they would like their baby if only circumstances were different.

The demand for termination sometimes comes from the partner or the parent. Although it is the woman who must make the decision, parents and partners need to be listened to since their opinion must influence the patient and decisions have to be made in the light of the total situation both emotional and practical. Parents and partners often have to be persuaded to look at the emotional as well as the practical issues.

Last year I saw a school teacher's wife who had two children. The youngest was now at school and she had started a part-time job so that to continue her pregnancy was a double blow to the family finances. Although she had always wanted more children she felt it sensible to stop at two. However, she had kept the baby equipment 'just in case'. She very much wanted to continue her pregnancy but felt her desire was not very sensible and her husband felt strongly that two was enough. I asked to see her husband. He too was being practical and sensible. He taught in the Education for Personal Relationships course at his school and was continually telling children that pregnancies must be the planned variety, so how could he accept any other sort? I felt that they both needed permission to indulge in a little irresponsible parenthood. The husband wrote to me later saying that he had been sceptical about attending for counselling. He thought they were two intelligent people who had made an intelligent decision, but during our discussion he had come to realise his wife's deep commitment to having this child and found that he too liked the idea of not having the make the 'sensible' decision. Regrettably solutions like this are not very common and when the woman wants her baby and her partner is equally sure that he does not the outcome is often resentment from her if she terminates and resentment from him if she does not, a climate that usually ensures that the relationship is not maintained.

Parents of very young girls may feel that they have the legal right to make the decision for their child. Sometimes, because she has not been asked, the girl has not told her parents that she wants to keep her baby. During counselling when her feelings and not just the practical situation are being looked at, she is able to express this wish and perhaps feels safer in expressing it in the presence of a third party. If the relationship between daughter and parents has not been good her pregnancy may be an expression of her search for love and affection. It may also be used as a weapon and expression of her resentment towards her parents. When a girl in this situation is told that her pregnancy will not be terminated unless she wants it done, she sometimes suddenly realises that the weapon she is wielding is a considerable threat to herself as well.

The really ambivalent patient is a great problem. As counselling proceeds, it becomes evident that it is a case of the emotional feelings versus the practical issues and if practical help can be offered this may tip the balance. Occasionally one meets a girl who has no strong feelings either way. She considers the issues as if she were buying a new sweater, makes her choice and then changes her mind about the colour.

Some patients make you behave like a practical doctor. You assess the size, tell them about the operation and make the arrangements. Others make you feel protective and maternal. You find yourself telling them they may ring you at home if they need you. Their return appointment is made sooner than usual so that you can make sure they are all right. Others make you angry and this interaction with the patient must be recognised and sometimes interpreted.

Pregnancy counselling must include some attempt to help the patient understand why her pregnancy occurred. Did she not recognise her need for contraception because she was unable to look at and accept her sexuality? Was she ignorant about contraception and where to get it? Was she frightened to seek help and was this due to a lack of confidence about her right to be sexual or fear of rejection? Whatever the cause, she now needs help in avoiding a recurrence and decisions about future contraception must be made before referral for termination.

If the decision about the pregnancy has been the right one there will be little counselling to be done later. If it has been the wrong one, I repeat, there is no second chance. Only an obligation to do the best you can in picking up the pieces.

Part VIII Hospital

This is a group of papers by doctors working in departments of gynaecology. Dr Blair was able to make a detailed study of the problems that lie behind requests for abortion, while the papers on work in antenatal and postnatal clinics and on receiving requests for sterilisation stress the need to maintain sensitivity under the pressure of a heavy work-load. Two further papers demonstrate the special contribution of a gynaecologist who is also a psychotherapist and a final paper describes the implications of emotional factors in genetic counselling.

31

Requests for termination of pregnancy

'I want an abortion doctor'

Margaret Blair

I wonder what sort of person comes to mind when you recall someone who has made that statement? Do you imagine a single girl whom you thinks regards abortion lightly as a method of birth control, or someone who has just been careless forgetting a few pills, or allowing her supply to run out? Perhaps like me you feel that it is not as simple as that.

How do you react? Have you strong views, for or against abortion, and do these views come across to your patients? Do you feel that anyone who gets pregnant, even accidently, really wants a baby? Or, are you able to listen and try to work out with the patient what lies behind her request?

By listening to a number of requests it soon becomes obvious that to understand what is going on two separate factors have to be considered: Why did the patient become pregnant at this time? Why is she asking for an abortion?

I am going to use some case histories to try to illustrate some of the points that I want to make.

Case Studies

Mrs A.

Mrs A, aged 40, was requesting termination for the second time. She had always had trouble with birth control but from time to time it became even more difficult and she either used it incorrectly or gave up altogether. She had four children and they were all doing well at school or university. The youngest was ten. During the interview she was very distressed and was crying. She said she certainly did not want any more children and the relationship with her husband was terrible — if she could leave him she would but it was not possible. He was lethargic and did not help her at all. He worked as a postman and she worked in an office.

By this time it was clear that this was an unusual family unit with both parents in quite ordinary jobs and the children already educated beyond the standard of their parents. I felt that Mrs A needed this to happen to supply something that was missing in her life and I got her to talk more about herself. Her family had broken up when she was very young and she had been brought up in homes. Her father was a bigamist. She went straight from that to say, with even more profuse tears, that 'he' had never married her — he did not think it was necessary. She felt it was another rejection but did not think she would marry him now even if he wanted to. This patient did not want another baby but she did want help for herself and with the relationship

196

with her partner and in her case both the pregnancy and the request for termination can be seen as an attempt to get this help.

She had the termination and returned two weeks later. She was much better and quite cheerful and said how relieved she felt. Even the relationship with her partner had improved. We discussed this and she was able to recognise that it was the stress of her personal problems and the problems with her partner that had caused her to misuse birth control and present her problems as an unwanted pregnancy. She is continuing to attend for follow-up at regular intervals.

Miss B.

Miss B. was 35 and came with a letter from her GP which stated that in his opinion she should have an abortion. He had known her since childhoold and the social and psychological circumstances made it unsuitable for her to continue the pregnancy. She had used a diaphragm and wondered why it should fail now. She was neatly but fairly plainly dressed and wore huge spectacles. At first she spoke without much feeling saying she had a very good job which she could not afford to give up. She had her own home on a mortgage and her 70-year-old mother lived with her. Her partner worked abroad and would not be returning for another four weeks. He was separated, waiting for a divorce and had no children. I said I was getting a picture of a background but did she know what she really wanted to do? She began to cry and the glasses had to come off. She said that until the week before she had been sure she should have an abortion but now she had some doubts. She felt she might not have another chance and might regret it in ten years time. She had arranged private ultrasound for herself two days previously and it had given her a shock when she had actually seen the baby. She had often wondered whether she was capable of getting pregnant and was pleased to find that she could. She wanted to tell her mother but would not do so if she decided on termination and she wanted to talk to her boy friend but had to wait for him to contact her. By this stage I had formed an early working relationship with her and we were able to talk about her uncertain femininity which she had had to test out by becoming pregnant. Although she wanted the baby she was not sure at that stage whether she could manage. It was left that she would return the next week.

[Unfinished.]

Miss C.

Miss C. was a 17-year-old Asian girl born and brought up in England. For several years she had been rebelling against her parents and extended family — a situation exaggerated by her confusion about the the two cultures in which she lived. She had become pregnant at 15 but the pregnancy was a hydatidiform mole and so there was no question of a baby to disgrace the family and no choice for her about whether the uterus should be evacuated. She was a bad attender for follow-up about the hydatidiform mole or anything else and her adolescent rebellion continued.

Two years later she was back again. This time it was a planned pregnancy and she said she really wanted the baby. She had run away from home twice and her family had had her traced by a private detective. She had gone to her boy friend — an unemployed West Indian in the Midlands. She was quite unable to get away from her mother who wanted to come into the interview with her and was insisting on an abortion. At first she would only whisper as she was afraid that her mother, who was not in the room with her, would hear. She reiterated how confused she was. She wanted the baby and they would not let her have it. She wanted to phone her boy friend but could not as she was never left alone.

She knew that in practical terms she should not have the baby and would have enormous difficulties if she did. We talked a lot about her confusion and how she felt she would hate her mother and aunt if she had the abortion but also her difficulty in cutting herself off emotionally from her family and her fear of doing this if she had the baby.

By the end of three interviews she could see the issues more clearly and was no longer saying that she had to have an abortion because of the family. She did however beg me to arrange something so that she could telephone her boy friend. I found myself arranging a ruse whereby she was admitted to a hospital bed and her mother sent home. When she had phoned her boy friend she left the hospital immediately.

[Unfinished.]

197

Mrs D.

Mrs D. was in her thirties and was a Roman Catholic using the safe period. She already had four boys. The first two were normal but the youngest two were haemophiliacs. She also came with a letter from her doctor strongly recommending an abortion which she agreed with when she first came with an eight-week pregnancy. She had very great difficulty with her youngest children as one or other has to attend hospital for bleeds nearly every day. She has a common-law husband but they are a close and supportive family unit.

She told me at the first visit that she did not like the idea of abortion but really felt she could not manage — it would not be right for the baby or the other children. With some doubts I arranged a termination but she did not turn up to have it done and so was asked to come for another interview. We went over everything again and talked about her fear that she would not be able to live with herself if she 'killed off the baby' but also her fear that she would really not manage if she had another haemophiliac . She was offered amniocentesis to sex the baby followed by foetoscopy to take some cord blood if it were a boy. By the end of the interview she said she would continue the pregnancy and not have any of the tests done — but of course that was not the end of the story. When she was in the obstetric department she wanted the baby at all costs but when she was in haematology with her children very distressed by their haemorrhages and injections she weakened again. She eventually decided to have amniocentesis, foetoscopy of a boy and termination of a haemophiliac. Fortunately, that was not necessary as it was a girl.

These cases are meant to demonstrate some of the circumstances in which patients who know quite well about birth control, misuse it. All could be said to be circumstances of increased stress and are used by a patient:

1. To draw attention to herself because of other problems, conscious or unconscious.
2. To draw attention to herself because of an unsatisfactory relationship with her partner. This is often a relationship which is just breaking up.
3. To demonstrate femininity by testing and proving fertility.
4. To express adolescent defiance where the struggle for independence from the parents is often more important than the relationship with the partner.

It must be apparent by now that in all these cases a relaxed and neutral doctor-patient relationship had to be established to allow the patients to express their feelings (if the doctor imposes attitudes or opinions, this process is interfered with and the patient can't gain the necessary insight into her situation). She can begin to consider in the same way why she is requesting an abortion. Again, these requests fall roughly into groups:

1. *Confrontation with reality.* A composite group of all the patients who have become pregnant for one of the above reasons and are now faced with the reality that they are going to have a baby and must consider all the practical problems that this will bring. Many are faced with the prospect of nowhere to live, no job and no other support, practical or emotional.
2. *Call for help with other problems.* There are some who use the termination clinic as an agent through which they can get help with other problems in their lives. Usually the termination clinic is not their first choice. Most would have liked to get help from parents, GPs psychiatrists or the law.
3. *Compliance with the wish of others.* Miss C., the Asian girl, is a very good example of this.
4. *Confirmation of the right to continue the pregnancy.* Miss B. and Mrs D.

And so, the patient who starts by saying 'I must have an abortion doctor' does not always mean it and it is the doctor's role to find out what she really means. If this is done the patients who eventually have an abortion may end up with mixed feelings of guilt, regret and relief, but will feel that they have made the right decision.

32

Detecting psychosexual problems in the antenatal clinic

James Bradshaw

The detection of psychosexual problems at the antenatal clinic does present an overwhelming problem and I am sure anyone who has worked in the cattle-market atmosphere of an NHS antenatal clinic would agree with me. There is a tremendous shortage of time. Patients rarely see the same doctor on two consecutive occasions and they are so busy looking after foetal well-being and for any signs of abnormal pregnancy that they are most unlikely to pick up the faint signals or even the fairly forceful signals of an anxious patient. Yet it may be possible by a small alteration in attitudes to prevent the onset of psychosexual disorders.

Cases can be divided into two categories: those with an existing psychosexual disorder, and those with a predisposition to psychosexual disorder.

Cases with an existing psychosexual disorder
The detection and management of these is not very different from the non-pregnant. It should be stressed however, that expectations of a cure with delivery are usually ill-founded. Vaginismus amounting to non-consummation is frequently unaffected by the passage of the foetal head down the birth canal. Indeed, I believe that cases of 'non-consummation' who succeed in becoming pregnant are more difficult to resolve, as the driving force has been removed. Vaginismus detected in the antenatal clinic is not usually improved after delivery.

Case Study

Rosemary
A small rather bossy school teacher, aged 29, was picked up as she had vaginismus when examined at the antenatal clinic at 36 weeks. She had no idea how she got pregnant, and seemed rather proud of the 'immaculate conception'. Examination during labour was difficult and she was delivered with forceps under general anaesthesia. She was referred to me by the obstetrician at her postnatal visit. Her husband was also a school teacher and looked a little like Hank Marvin. He was 34. She was an only child. Her mother was very strait-laced and the boss of her family. She switched off the television if there was any sex scene, never talked to Rosemary about sex, but did to her surprise explain about menses. Rosemary had never masturbated, and never attempted intercourse before marriage. The first vaginal examination she suffered was by a doctor who said 'If you are like this

with me, you can't be much good to your husband'. She was told her vagina was too small by another doctor and given dilators. She had seen a psychiatrist several times, who told her to imagine intercourse with Paul, her husband.

She taught tiny infants and needed to be in control. She certainly controlled me successfully, and I found myself attempting a one-finger vaginal examination with her lying on her side as 'it was better like that'. The moment of truth was not illuminating. She was tight-lipped and long-suffering, but did not drop her guard and give me any of her feelings. She had no memory of childbirth at all and had not breastfed and she was now fostering her child so she could go to work. There was not much femininity about her; she was an efficient rather than a loving mother. She thought of men as walking companions and her happiest days had been spent youth hostelling.

It was not easy to get her to betray any inner feelings, and we were frequently side-tracked, so that I could not find out much about her inner personality. I suggested that control was important in her job, and that this was carried to the bedroom. Would she be able to have intercourse on top of her husband? That would be rather embarrassing. She resisted self-examination initially, but then undertook it in the way her school class might examine a biological specimen under instruction.

I sensed as the weeks went by that she was as disenchanted with me as she had been with her psychiatrist. She pretended, at least that was my feeling, that things were improving. Indeed she said they had nearly made it once, but the poor chap had ejaculated prematurely. But finally she failed to attend. Her GP congratulated me when he saw me next, saying Rosemary had told him everything was fine. I did not believe it, and later the GP confirmed that I was right. She had opted out yet again. There was certainly no improvement in her symptoms after childbirth, and perhaps she will succeed in conceiving again without being penetrated.

Cases with a predisposition to psychosexual disorder
Can we obtain clues to warning signs that a patient is going to lose her libido?

The patient's expectations are important. These vary enormously from patient to patient as does the attitude of the husband. The patient who has read all about natural childbirth and believes that she will sail through her delivery may be more devastated psychologically by a traumatic confinement than another who is more apprehensive. Hopefully pregnancy is associated with a spontaneous delivery, the husband is present and supportive during the first and second stages, breastfeeding is established with bonding and the family unit is happy as a result. Reality may, however, be very different.

Obstetricians today are striving to make the art of midwifery into an exact science and a patient may be given a date on which she makes her body over to the staff of the maternity unit. She finds herself shaved, starved and monitored in a rather alarming way. She may have a normal delivery, but at any deviation from normal, assisted instrumental delivery or Caesarean section is performed. Breastfeeding may not be possible and perineums can be sore from episiotomy or tears.

At the antenatal clinic a few questions were 'slipped in' during the booking visit about the patient's feelings about sex, pregnancy and motherhood.

A past history was taken as a routine, but the patient was also questioned regarding her emotions and feelings. Any resultant fears were recorded. A previous termination can make a baby even more precious. The grief of a past stillbirth can be reawakened by a new pregnancy. Particular note was taken of prolonged labour, forceps, perineal tears with post-partum soreness.

Nearly every mother has unspoken fears about her unborn child, or her own ability to stand up to the stress of delivery. These questions were deliberately structured so that they were not time-consuming, to evaluate what could reasonably be achieved in a busy clinic.

Occasionally we found that the wife did not wish her husband to be present, perhaps to preserve some mystery of her body. I have yet to see a woman who can remain mysterious or sophisticated whilst bearing down. When the husband did not want to attend, it was seen as a signpost to lack of union in the family.

The impression I have, and it cannot be supported by figures, is that amongst psychosexual patients there is a relatively low incidence of breastfeeders. Some women were embarrassed by sexual arousal when they fed their babies and guilty when they experienced sexual pleasures. This is a point I try to explain to mothers in advance, and my midwives are aware of this possible problem.

'Do you intend to breastfeed?' The way the question was answered was of particular interest. A thoughtful 'No' or a 'No' based on previous failure was accepted as normal. An aggressive 'No' which on occasions was accompanied by involuntary flexion of the forearms across the chest could be significant.

Less frequent and less enjoyable sexual intercourse during the antenatal period, followed by post-partum abstinence, perhaps prolonged by perineal damage or long-lasting lochia, alters the sexual habit. Where the frequency of intercourse fell, the reason was explored. It was not uncommon for sex to occur less often because the husband was afraid of damaging the baby. In these cases the wife could be irritated, frustrated and resentful.

Vaginal examination

It is not always prudent to perform an internal examination at first booking, if for example, there has been previous miscarriage. However, when performed it once again was of proved value, and was responsible for uncovering psychosexual cases.

Case Studies

Mrs T. W.

Mrs T. W., aged 20, had been married for two years. She was very defensive at the booking clinic; she emphatically refused to breastfeed. Neither did *she* want her husband present at delivery.

It was her first pregnancy and I sensed instant hostility which I challenged. She said she hated seeing doctors, and had never been ill. Her replies were monosyllabic and most discouraging. Her brittle antagonism broke, however, when a vaginal examination was attempted. She was terrified of labour, and sure that there was no room for the baby as intercourse had always been painful. She actually smiled when I acknowledged her fears, and there was a marked change in the whole character of the interview.

She was one of four siblings. Her mother had told her that sex was dirty and that she had not had sex with her father for years. When Theresa was 16 she was raped in the back of a car, and vividly remembers the pain of having a rough youth pushing his fingers into her vagina.

Sex had always been very painful, and she was sure that she had been damaged. We talked about labour and relaxation; she accepted self-examination and during the pregnancy the vaginismus improved. She had a spontaneous vaginal delivery with an episiotomy. There was a recurrence of her vaginismus at the postnatal clinic when I saw her. She rapidly responded to treatment and after two further visits felt that everything was now fine and she did not need to return.

Mrs T. C. G.

Mrs T. C. G., aged 21, was a rather dowdy woman, with heavy eyebrows and a reticent manner. She was very nervous at her first visit when she was already 36 weeks pregnant and I saw her for the first time. It was a busy clinic and I had little time to talk to her, but I noted she had some vaginismus. Her husband was away at the time she expected her baby. She intended to try and breastfeed, though she thought she would have problems and her breasts were small.

I do not honestly think I handled her very well at this point as the pressures of a large clinic, when my colleague was away, did not encourage me to uncover a problem. However, I noted that I would like to see her next time, and booked her for the end of the clinic.

At this interview she admitted that when eight years of age her father had molested her twice. He had pushed her back on the bed and laid his penis on her, but not penetrated her. She had cried on the first occasion and been sent to buy sweets. The second time she told her mother and all hell was let loose. As a result she had never been allowed to be alone with her father, though they had been close previously. She felt rejected by the family.

She had never masturbated or had sex before marriage. Intercourse was occasionally sore and she never enjoyed it and could not touch her husband's penis. I discussed labour, and after a while she became less agitated, and she was not acutely anxious about the delivery. She proved to be difficult to examine during labour, and ultimately was delivered with the ventouse. However, she is enjoying motherhood, though she breastfed only whilst in hospital.

I feel that she missed out, in that she was not identified as having a problem at first booking, and when she was found to need help, it was in the middle of a busy antenatal clinic. I hope that we have since recovered lost ground, as she is still attending and seems to be improving.

Mrs V. L.

Mrs V. L. was a plump, busy 30 year old. She helped run a youth hostel and was quick to answer questions and jumped on the couch when she was asked. She had been married for three years. Her two previous pregnancies consisted of a termination in 1974, when she had virtually been raped following a casual meeting in a pub, and then a miscarriage in 1980. Her family and husband were unaware of the termination.

She did not want to breastfeed as she would not have the time with all the work she had in the youth hostel. Her husband, she thought, would be present at delivery. Examination was painful and mild vaginismus present. She admitted that intercourse was sore, she had never been orgasmic and her libido, since becoming pregnant, was very low.

She appeared to be very guilty about the termination, and admitted that her 'rape' had really been quite exciting. This point appeared to be the key to her problems, and I managed to get her to discuss her feelings of guilt.

Recently she had an uneventful delivery of a 7 lb 2 oz boy. At the postnatal clinic she was, surprisingly, still breastfeeding her baby. Since this visit she has had successful intercourse, orgasmically on one occasion, and was looking very happy when I last saw her.

I feel that in her case, the warning alert was in her past history. The vaginismus was mild and could well have been unremarked. The reluctance to breastfeed was an added factor.

Summary

Existing psychosexual problems rarely improve with pregnancy, and it is a false hope to expect vaginismus to be cured mechanically by a physiological Fenton's operation.

Of greater interest to me is the possibility of tilting the questioning and therapy of a pregnant woman towards the emotions, making sure that during the fuss over the baby, these are not overlooked, and the husband is brought out of his shadowy role and included in the family unit. It takes little extra time to ask just a few more questions at the antenatal booking clinic, and it can alert me to patients' fears and unmask the sexually inadequate, so that appropriate support can be offered.

A mothercraft class, likewise, can discuss the emotional changes in the coming alteration to the simple one-to-one relationship before delivery. (In co-operation with our midwife tutor, a session is devoted to exploring emotional changes with the expectant mothers. This at least ensures that emotional changes could be expected, and we hoped might prepare mothers for any difficulties.) Having prepared the ground, patients in difficulties will be more ready to confess them at the postnatal clinic.

I see no reason why every maternity unit should not be reorientated in this way.

33

Psychosexual problems seen in the postnatal clinic

Elizabeth J. Deman

The postnatal visit comprises the final chapter in the saga of pregnancy and labour. The interview is structured according to a standardised pattern; previous methods of birth control are discussed and the method the patient now wants to use for contraception is established. Sexual problems can easily be missed and overlooked because the patient presents with physical complaints and expects a physical cure. It is extremely rare for example to hear a frank complaint about loss of libido. However, the following should alert the doctor that this patient may have a sexual problem.

First, the appearance of the patient: the manner in which she enters the consulting room; how she manages her baby and perhaps a sibling during the interview. Second, when taking the history you may hear how she has not slept a wink since the birth, vaginal bleeding has never ceased, she still has profuse discharge or backache. She may complain about a painful perineum, shooting pains up the vagina or lower abdominal pain. Third, difficulties may not be suspected until just prior to the physical examination. Comments such as 'Please be careful doctor, I do not think you will be able to examine me. I seem to have been stitched up too tightly'. Or 'You can see the lump there that prevents examination. The stitches are still very sore. There is a tender spot just inside the vagina'. All such comments should alert the doctor to the patient's anxieties. She may, in the privacy of the examination couch, be able to confess that penetration is impossible, that she and her husband have tried several times to have intercourse since the birth and it has been quite impossible.

Case Studies

'Mother-earth'

A young woman in her early thirties caused chaos on her way into the consulting room. Sister had innocently tried to help by picking up the carry-cot with the new baby in it while mother struggled with her elder son who was scrambling in and out of a pushchair. The boy was attached by a long rope to mother's hand. As soon as Sister attempted to lift the carry-cot the little boy screamed and his mother said 'Put it down at once, you see Johnny has never seen his sister handled by anybody else but mummy and daddy'. When eventually some kind of calm had been restored all the participants were anxious to get the consultation and examination over with as quickly as possible.

Good 'Mother Earth' had been a biology teacher in her youth, and was therefore familiar with the process of reproduction. She succumbed to examination and refitting of her IUD with resignation, and I was only too conscious of monumental problems, but refrained from delving beneath the surface. Despite all that, she did feel able to come back six weeks later to have her coil checked. She came in looking very smart and well groomed and told me she had been able to leave her toddler at home. He had got chickenpox and daddy was looking after him. She clearly wanted the opportunity to tell me how she felt. There were many reasons why she was so tense and totally ill-at-ease on the first occasion; but it was nice that she felt she could come back knowing she would find somebody who was prepared to listen to her difficulties.

Gillian

The second patient whose history I would like to share with you is Gillian, aged 35, who makes costumes for films. She came in depressed and looking as though she was about to burst into tears. She was actually a pleasant presentable woman who had regained her figure and was well groomed. She talked all the time and her only real initial complaint was that of constipation. In fact she was so preoccupied with this that a prescription for suppositories was written out before continuing with the consultation. In response to discussing the fitting of an intra-uterine device, which had been recommended on the ward, she told me that her marriage was a total farce. All her time was taken up in looking after Kathy, the new baby. She felt tired, in fact there had been no sex since prior to her marriage. She discovered she was pregnant on the day of her wedding and this turned her right off sex. They had a belated honeymoon which in her words was a 'total disaster'. She feels lumpy and unattractive and hated herself when pregnant. She and her husband, who works on films, had known each other 18 months prior to marriage and had lived together for five months before deciding to marry. In fact he had been the one who was so keen to get married. She had had difficulty in committing herself to 'losing her freedom' as she put it. She also talked of a nervous breakdown after her mother's death.

She readily agreed to having an intra-uterine device fitted and was asked to get up on the couch. Somehow I expected to see a scarred abdomen. This feeling must have come from the patient and was so strong that when I did examine her nice smooth stomach, quite free of stretch marks with excellent muscle tone, I told the patient how I had expected to see a scar and that these feelings of a damaged body must have come from her. Immediately she changed the topic and we found ourselves discussing breastfeeding which she said she would like to give up because Kathy did not seem to be getting enough and she had felt confused by the instructions of the health visitor. I found myself discussing this as another mother. It was difficult for the doctor and patient to get back to sex at all. You do not normally discuss sex with your mother anyway. The coil was fitted without any difficulty. The physical examination was very clinical and emotionless but she seemed very keen to return for a further prolonged consultation the following week. Again she arrived extremely well groomed, her hair prettily done. She had a sun tan and admitted that she felt a great deal less tired.

In this case the feeling for the need of a mother figure to help her through the first few weeks post-partum was so strong that I succumbed to her request of looking after her needs.

Mrs X.

This case illustrates the therapeutic value of the vaginal examination. Mrs X. came for her postnatal, free of complaints. She had taken the pill for years prior to this pregnancy and wanted to restart as soon as she finished breastfeeding. Her husband and she had decided that they would use the sheath till then. It was not until she undressed and was preparing for examination that there was any clue that something was amiss. She quite calmly told me once she was up on the couch that she was afraid that I would not be able to examine her down below, and enquired, 'Is it normal to be stitched up too tightly and for it to take some months before penetration is possible?' She and her husband had tried several times but it just was not possible: 'It was quite different down there since the birth.' They had had a marvellous sex life for seven years before they had planned their first baby. This discovery after the birth had been a terrible shock to them both.

I looked at the perineum and asked her to show me where she had closed up. She put her finger in the vulval area rather hesitantly. She was very embarrassed and did not want to go on. Very gently

206

I inserted one finger and then two fingers. She flushed up and her lips trembled and she tearfully told me how she still sometimes wakes up screaming in the middle of the night and sees that big black doctor taking off his white coat, rolling up his sleeves, putting on his gloves and putting his hand and arm right up inside her, telling the midwife that it should not be long before she is fully dilated. Mrs X. shudderingly felt that he had plunged his examining hand right into the pit of her stomach. Her only other recollection of the birth was waiting for the student to stitch her up. The first stitching had to be undone after argument between the midwife and houseman. She felt as though she had been there for hours before she was eventually cleaned up and returned to her bed. It took about two minutes for the patient to say all this. As soon as she had said it, she said 'Oh, I'm so glad I've told you. The horror of it'. I just listened and then I asked her if she would check for herself how it felt down there now, now that I had been able to feel. She got off the couch, we squatted down together and I guided her to the vulval area because clearly she had never actually explored her own vagina during all her married life. It was a great revelation to discover where her vagina went to and where it ended. She did not talk about it but just smiled and seemed very pleased with herself. Her worst fears had been dispelled — she was entirely reassured and keen to return to her husband and share her relief with him.

The anxieties and fears about what may have happened to the perineum, vagina and even cervix during delivery can sometimes be dispelled very quickly during the examination.

As in all other clinical situations the doctor must try to make a diagnosis from the history and examination. If the patient is obviously seriously depressed, therapy is beyond the scope of this clinic and psychiatric referral is indicated. This is very rare because severe puerperal depression comes on earlier than six weeks post-partum. If the sexual problem seems to be highlighted by the recent pregnancy but is long-standing a contract of an agreed number of sexual counselling sessions may be arranged. If the problem stems from the recent pregnancy and labour, skilful use of the vaginal examination can often avert a chronic problem.

Many mothers have read far more books on the subject of producing babies than many of us know about, know exactly what the perfect, beautiful childbirth is going to be like, and when they end up with an epidural and perhaps a lower segment Caesarian section they feel terribly let down.

We may perhaps consider pain as an expression of anger or associate tears with frustration. If the patient is able to let go, release her feelings and feel free to share them with the doctor, she will then be able to return to her husband and share her pre-pregnancy sexual desires with him.

Sexual problems can easily be missed. The patient expects solutions to physical problems. However, sensitive recognition of the woman's needs and feelings at the time of interview and examination can avert months of subsequent misery and counselling.

34

Psychosexual problems revealed during medical consultation requesting sterilisation

James Bradshaw

As an Army gynaecologist I see wives and families of service personnel. I felt it might be of interest to go through the records of my first hundred female psychosexual consultations and discover how many problems arose in those who had undergone either hysterectomy or sterilisation. None of the 66 patients under 30 years old had been sterilised.

Among the group of 34 older women one of the five patients complaining of orgasmic dysfunction had been sterilised but she did not attribute her symptoms to the operation. Of the 29 'unresponsive' patients over 31, 13 had been sterilised either by tubal ligation or hysterectomy. The symptoms of seven of these patients dated from the time of operation. It had been hoped that in four other cases psychosexual problems could have improved with operation. I also noted that one patient dated her symptoms from her husband's vasectomy and that two thought extensive infertility investigations had put them off sex.

Two case studies illustrate the importance of *pre*-operative counselling.

Case Studies

Mrs C.

Mrs C., a corporal's wife was referred by her GP with a request for sterilisation. She was a cheerful, talkative, dark-haired little Geordie. She had made up her mind that she did not want any more children. She was 28 and had one daughter, Karen. Her husband was in the waiting room and I decided to leave him there until she had talked a while longer.

She had been married two years and since her child was born could not bear her husband to touch her. The childbirth itself had been uneventful and she had refused to breastfeed (this with a distasteful look). She did not believe in the pill, her husband would not use the sheath and the thought of having anything inside her was so revolting it made her sick when she had been shown the cap and the coil. Needless to say, tampons could not be inserted. She looked quite shocked when I asked her if she masturbated, and very shocked when I suggested she might like to examine her own vagina. It seemed almost inevitable that examination was impossible as she was menstruating.

She blurted out smiling shamefully that there was another child born about a year before she was married to Brian. At first she kept the child, but then decided to have him adopted. Brian offered to

208

have him, but 'No, that wasn't right'. She did feel guilty now, but felt it had been all for the best.

She had had sex before marriage, but only the father of her adopted child had given her an orgasm. He had gone off to Germany and had not been interested when she said she was pregnant.

Her mother had died of tuberculosis when she was two, leaving her and her one elder sister with her father. He had hanged himself in the kitchen six months later, and been found by her sister who never talked about it. Her maternal grandparents had looked after her until she was seven. When they died she was taken in by her paternal grandparents, but never got on with them. This grandfather died of cancer and the grandmother took to drink, often having to be brought home by neighbours. She had gone to London to work, but became very depressed and took an overdose of Valium. She did not think she had really wanted to end it all, really she just wanted to be noticed.

She lived with her sister when she had her first baby, but had to leave as the husband was very violent and used to hit her. Once he attacked the sister with a knife and threw her downstairs.

This, I assure you, was unprompted information. Suddenly I recalled that Brian was sitting in the waiting room and thought we had better have him in. He was a very normal looking man, the sort one would have trouble describing to the police. He talked freely, did not call me Sir too often or stand to attention, which I find inhibiting, and agreed that they did have sex problems, or rather that *she did*.

I was still a bit dazed from the potted history of her life, but collected what was left of my wits. I would not even contemplate sterilising his wife until we had worked through the sexual problems and frankly was not too sure I would agree even then. I added a few platitudes about mutual pleasuring and patience, and hoped he did not feel excluded, which in fact he had been. At this point I definitely felt that sterilisation would be an unmitigated disaster. She seemed intent on rejecting motherhood completely and was very insecure in looking after her child.

I have seen her five times since. We eventually did get round to examining her, though I had to desist the first time as I thought she was going to vomit, she was so upset. She was surprised that it was not nasty in there and even agreed to examine herself.

As we talked I tried to show her that her sterilisation request was caused by her difficulty in accepting her role as a mother. She had felt guilty in allowing her first baby to be adopted and often felt angry with Karen. She regretted that she had not breastfed her daughter and bonding was minimal.

Her enjoyment of sex improved and she became orgasmic. She suggested that she was sufficiently confident as a wife and mother not to see me again, and there was no mention at all of sterilisation when she left.

Mrs H.

Mrs H., aged 38, had been married 14 years to a divorcee who was a civil engineer in the City. They came together referred by their GP for sterilisation. David did not feel too confident about vasectomy and she was quite happy to have the operation. They had three children, a son of 18 from his first marriage and two daughters of 11 and eight.

She was a very cold woman and sat bolt upright. I asked her if she was a schoolteacher. No, a telephone-operator supervisor. A very responsible job and she had to keep her wits about her. He was very quiet and reasonable, but not impressive. He was 15 years older than Sheila and his first wife had gone off with a younger man. He had married Sheila within 18 months. His mother, who also worked in the telephone exchange, had brought her home and introduced them. They had married and lived in his mother's house until she had died a few years before.

Sex — well, they had it; rather as they took the *Sunday Telegraph* it appeared. He sometimes could not get an erection, and with her cold exterior I was not surprised. That was why he did not want a vasectomy — in case it made him worse. She had never liked sex and had never had sex with anyone else. I asked her if she would come back and see me and she agreed, if I thought it would do any good.

She came alone next time and sat down with a cold, bold front daring me to extract any warmth from the situation. I temporarily passed and took a history of her family hoping that something, anything, might appear as a sign of warmth.

Her mother was forever in her house. Her father had died of bronchopneumonia the year before and she felt very afraid of old age. She had drifted into marriage, never really enjoyed sex and only had an orgasm if she masturbated alone. Her honeymoon in Jersey had been good, but she came home to her mother-in-law's house and everything was in apple-pie order. Her parents had always encouraged her to be a sensible only child. There was little affection and she could not remember ever being cuddled.

She did not know why she could masturbate herself but had no feelings when her husband tried. We talked about vulnerability and relaxation, of sharing all of ourselves with our partner. I saw her on a number of occasions, but never broke down the cold exterior she consistently presented. She had no need, it seemed, of a sexual relationship and her marriage was happy. She was prepared to satisfy her husband by letting him insert his penis, and he was not complaining.

I am afraid I agreed to sterilise her eventually and saw her twice afterwards. It will come as no surprise to any of you that she is unchanged sexually.

35

Care of patients with a known abnormal foetus

Frank Johnson

In medicine, new techniques are continuously becoming available which solve specific problems but may produce other problems. These secondary problems, if left unsolved, limit the real benefits of the new techniques. Ultrasound is now used widely within obstetrics, having innumerable benefits. The patient I wish to present to you, however, demonstrates an unavoidable complication of the new technique. This case is a means of illustrating and discussing the management of patients with a known abnormal foetus.

Case Study

This patient was a 35-year-old primigravida with an 11-year history of infertility, caused by endometriosis which was diagnosed by laparoscopy and had responded to Danazol. After the endometriosis had resolved, ovulation had been stimulated by the use of Clomid. There was also a poor sperm count in her husband. In July 1980 she was pregnant and scanning revealed twins. She was offered blood test for serum alpha foeto-protein levels. She had a high level, even for twins. Aminocentesis was attempted from both sacs but the levels found were normal and presumably, therefore, both taken from the same sac. Scanning at a slightly later stage clearly showed that one twin was an anencephalic foetus. She was told about this while I was away on holiday.

After my holiday I asked her to come and see me. She had been very pleased that she was pregnant and was almost overwhelmed by the fact that she was having twins. Now, I explained to her that I thought her situation might be difficult to accept and cope with and I asked her to talk about how she felt. It had taken her some time to get used to being pregnant and to the fact that she was going to have twins. She was delighted — she felt she was making up for her years of infertility. During the first session she talked at length of her feelings of extreme hurt and felt that life was very unfair to her. When she was told that one twin was abnormal it felt like being stabbed in the back with a knife. She was unable to think about her future children, unable to buy any clothes. She had been advised to think about the normal child and forget about the abnormal one and this was precisely what she could not do. She was having difficulty talking with her husband who was obviously equally hurt and saddened by the events. She felt and looked depressed. She was basically an intelligent, warm, out-going person. When people asked her 'How are the twins?' she found it extremely difficult to explain that she was only going to get one child at the end of it all. A few interpretations were made such as that she was stuck in the pain and was preferring to withdraw herself from people and pain. Towards the end of the interview she expressed her appreciation of having the opportunity to talk. She then asked how much of the head was going to be present. She had looked at the picture on the scanner but could not make much of it out. She began also exploring her fantasies and fears of the deformity and her feelings of incompetence as a woman. I felt a considerable degree of pain for her difficulty.

About a week later she said she felt very much better, as if she had been thoroughly analysed and had been sorry for herself in the past. She was now able to think about and even look at clothes for the normal child. She had gone home and talked until the early hours of the morning with her husband. She had cried and still felt depressed and sad. It was worse when she was alone and she was apprehensive about leaving work in the near future. She accused me of avoiding giving her details of the anencephalic child but I simply said 'Do you think it is I who was reluctant to talk about this?' She immediately replied, 'Well no, I suppose it was really me'. I asked her if she would like to look at a photograph of an anencephalic child, but she said 'No, I'm not yet ready for that'.

The further three sessions were at weekly intervals. She made significant progress. She became less depressed and was communicating much better with her husband and friends and neighbours. She repeatedly asked for details about the abnormal child but always declined seeing a photograph. She saw the abnormal child on the scanner, which was rather like seeing through a glass dimly. She expressed some resentment at being told so early in pregnancy that she had an abnormal child, but also felt that it would have been extremely difficult to be suddenly presented with an abnormal child at delivery.

At about 29 weeks she was admitted to the ward for routine bed rest. I agreed to see her when she was in the ward if she felt she needed to be seen and we would not meet again for about three weeks. I had no request from her but after three weeks she found herself in some difficulties. She always felt reluctant to talk with me, felt that she should be able to cope by herself and yet she was grateful for the opportunity to talk. The patient in the next bed was also having twins in an unwanted fourth pregnancy. She found it impossible to sleep in the next bed to this patient. The feelings of unfairness, pain and hurt came back very strongly and she was moved by the Ward Sister into a single room. Initially she found it difficult to hear the other children crying but eventually became more interested in the children around her. She was seen at about two-weekly intervals. On one occasion her fears were of one twin dominating the other, particularly that the abnormal twin would take all the nutrition, etc., from the normal twin. Regular scanning showed that both twins were growing and from this she obtained considerable reassurance. During the time I had to play two roles. First, to allow her to fantasise, to explore and work through some of her anxieties. Second, I had to function on a more direct, organic level and to answer in a direct way some of her fears, and to discuss some of the complications which twin pregnancies can develop and how these can be overcome. Ultrasound was used in a positive way to relieve her anxieties. I also felt that her husband was being left out and she asked him if he wished to see me. He did not. She thought that he felt as long as she was all right, he was all right. Around Christmastime she found it extremely difficult. She could not go into a party of relatives and be happy with the other children.

When she was 38 weeks she was induced using prostaglandin pessaries. Labour developed easily and progress in the first stage was rapid and uneventful. Delivery was supervised by a midwife. I attended the delivery as an observer and as a director. Her husband was there too. The first twin was the normal child. During this delivery her reactions were warm and positive. She touched the baby's head as it was delivered and was given the child to cuddle.

Through the delivery of the second child neither she nor her husband wished to see or touch the child. I deliberately delayed removing the abnormal child for a few minutes to see if their attitude changed. The child was then taken out into the sluice. The parish priest came in after he had baptized the normal child and touched her, which visibly shook her and both husband and wife gripped hands together. I asked her how she was feeling and she said 'OK, but a little shaken'. When I went out to the changing room I met her husband. We were both caught together literally with our trousers down! I was placed in a dilemma. To say nothing seemed to be extremely false but to talk might be interpreted as putting pressure on him to talk. I risked the latter course. He spoke for about 40 minutes and during all that time he gave two impressions: that he wished to talk, and that he wished to stop talking and get out. He felt he had lost a son. In whatever form or shape they had come, the babies were still his sons and it had been very painful to him. He had lost his father some nine months previously and found the day's events difficult to cope with. Some of his previous feelings were recurring at that moment. He had coped with his father's loss by walking his dog on the beach and it was only some three or four days later that the events struck him. I asked if he felt I had pushed him into talking about the day's events, but he said 'No, no. I wanted to talk. We wouldn't have been able to get through these last few months without your assistance'. I invited him to come back and talk again if he wanted, but he has never returned.

The next day the anencephalic child was still alive and I arranged for the mother to come and see me again in my office. She said she felt 'fine', a little sad, particularly when she was feeding the normal child, because somehow he had been deprived of a brother and companion. She felt it was a bit hard that the abnormal child had lived so long. I asked if either she or her husband had seen the abnormal child but neither of them had done so. I then said, unfortunately, 'Most people who do not see their abnormal child regret it later'. I was feeling like bursting and was completely aware of her avoidance of the pain, but I could not put the feeling clearly into an interpretive observation. Immediately I had said those words, I regretted them. She replied with some anger that she still did not wish to see the abnormal child and wished to forget about him and get on with enjoying and looking after the normal one. She enquired about funeral arrangements. Was it they or the hospital who would make these arrangements? I felt it would be strongly advisable for them to organise the funeral arrangements themselves and suggested this. The husband talked to the undertaker, vicar, etc., which he found very difficult. She did not go to the funeral. On two further occasions in the postnatal ward she said she regretted not going to the funeral because she was not there to comfort her husband, who had found the experience 'brutal'. During the immediate postnatal period she said she felt on 'Cloud 9', delighted she had a normal child but a little afraid of going back to 'reality' at home. We agreed she would not be seen again unless she requested it, except at the postnatal visit to discuss the question of sterilisation. I was not willing to make arrangements for sterilisation at this point but would discuss it later. She was discharged home on the eighth day.

Four days after she was discharged she asked to see me, and came simply to say how right I had been. As soon as she went home she intensely regretted not having seen the abnormal child. She felt guilty that she had rejected one of the children 'without a glance'. She was now feeling a little better but was still depressed and crying a great deal. She imagined while feeding the normal child that there were two normal children. I made the interpretation that she was still unable to accept the fact that she had had an abnormal child. During that session I felt progress had been satisfactory.

About six weeks later I sent an appointment for postnatal check. She came in rather surprised to get it. Things were rough. She was still depressed but beginning to improve. I felt a very severe control in the patient. She had been talking to her GP about how she felt and the GP had said 'What is the problem? You've got one child. In any case, if I were delivering you, you wouldn't have had the chance of seeing the abnormal child'. I was then aware of the strong negative feelings she had towards me. She wished I had forced her to look at the abnormal child or not to look at it although she admitted that she would not have liked me to have done this. She had seen a film on TV about abnormal children; one was an anencephalic child but a woollen hat had been placed over the defect. She wished she had seen this film before her delivery. At this point I pointed out to her that, first, she had some anger and resentment towards me and was having difficulty in expressing it, and, second, she was still unable to accept the fact that she had had an abnormal child. She accepted these interpretations and went on to discuss the sterilisation, saying her husband was quite keen on having the operation but she did not wish either of them to be sterilised just now. It was too final and in any case she was really wanting another child. She added, 'I'm not sure if I'm wanting to replace the one I've lost'. Intercourse had also been painful, which confused her. She thought it might be due to using the sheath or to the fact that the episiotomy scar had not satisfactorily healed. However, her GP had examined her and told her that all was well. I made the interpretation that intercourse had not much pleasure for her at the moment. It had previously resulted in a very painful pregnancy, etc. These interpretations she three-quarters accepted. She still partly felt that it was purely organic but also recognised that the pain could be related to her emotional turmoil. She had some resentment towards her husband. He had said that she would not have been able to cope with two if she had had two. She added 'If I was going to feel the way I am feeling now I couldn't have coped with them'. She felt isolated. I suggested her difficulty in expressing her resentment towards me was similar to her inability to deal with her anger and resentment towards her husband. There was a considerable degree of self-criticism, anger, etc. We discussed another appointment and she said 'Well, let's see what happens, but I would quite like to see you again after a month's time'.

I told her she found it very difficult to accept any help because of her strong belief that she should be able to cope with these situations herself. I saw her again after a month. She seemed infinitely better. Only very occasionally had she been troubled. She had even been able to see other mothers with twins without being disturbed. She was not preoccupied with the loss. Intercourse was now enjoyable. Her child was sleeping better and relations with her husband were back to normal. She was on the mini-pill and felt quite satisfied about that form of contraception. She did not wish to come back again but I left an open invitation to see me at any time.

This case demonstrates several valuable points. Ultrasound enables the diagnosis of an abnormal foetus to be made early in pregnancy. This is a very recent possibility. If an abnormal foetus is diagnosed a decision for termination can usually also be made early in the pregnancy. The technique therefore presents patients and staff with acute emotional conflicts at an earlier stage in pregnancy than would have been possible in the past. If there had been a single pregnancy in this case it would have been easier for the patient to work through her feelings. After delivery this patient said she was glad she had been informed early about the abnormal child and felt that it would have been a terrible shock to be presented with an abnormal child at delivery. She had, as it were, 20 weeks to begin the process of mourning. However, this process was complicated by the fact that the abnormal child was still alive inside her and she was also going to have one normal child. Resolution of these conflicts has, I feel, not been completely achieved to the present date, but was made easier by the fact that one person was handling both aspects of her management. There was a very fine line between her realistic fears and her fantasies. It was, I think, important that she could explore her fantasies without having the process blocked off by immediate simple advice. At the time I felt that she needed, after exploring some of her fantasies, concrete advice. If she had seen separately a pure psychotherapist and an organic specialist, I think it is quite possible she would have been confused about which of her conflicts were organic, and to be discussed with the organic specialist, and which were emotional, to be discussed with the psychotherapist. In other words, she was enabled to explore her fantasies with more freedom and resolve her anxieties to a great degree precisely because one person was managing both of her conditions.

There are real difficulties doing psychotherapy and organic work together but there are also real advantages. A great number of patients have virtually only organic problems but even in these there is always some anxiety. There are other patients who have virtually only psychological problems. But, there is also another group of patients who have both psychological and organic problems simultaneously and one person handling both conditions can be of great assistance provided that person is aware of what is taking place in each different situation. Modifications of the management of this couple were made as a result of dealing with both aspects of the wife's condition, e.g. waiting to remove the abnormal child from the labour ward and delaying discussing or agreeing to do a sterilising operation.

Conclusion

Without any apologies I wish to be provocative. I would like the Institute to move into handling more of these emotional problems within obstetrics and gynaecology. Personally, I think the title of the Institute is open to a narrow interpretation of what psychosexual means. If it is perceived as only being related to and involved with the act of intercourse, then some of these problems I have been discussing may not be relevant to the Institute's work. If a wider interpretation is held, then these problems naturally fall into the Institute's work. In the past, in my view, the teaching of gynaecology has almost ignored the fact that emotions play an important part in the problems of our speciality and they need to be recognised and management integrated with the organic part of our work. I would hope that in the future the Institute would assist at all stages in the training of gynaecologists.

214

36

Emotional problems associated with infertile patients

Frank Johnson

In my routine gynaecological clinic, a patient was referred to me who complained of sub-fertility. She had been married for eight years. Except for some mild obesity no abnormality was detected. When I explained this to her I felt within her a very high degree of anxiety. She said 'If I become pregnant now, I am not sure if I really want the baby or not. I am not sure if I can cope with a baby but I am now nearly 35 and realise I haven't much more time left'. I felt we should go into the matter more fully. The first session took place about six weeks later. She said again that she wanted a baby but was frightened to hold babies. She was extremely worried about the pain in labour. Intercourse was never very good, but just acceptable. She was tense and I was beginning to feel tense and tight. She said she was always a shy person and had a strict and secluded upbringing, brought up by her grandparents because her mother had died when she was eight years old. Her father was a postman and she felt that he could not look after her because he had to get up early in the mornings. I asked her about nervous problems in her past life. After her grandparents died she had been put on tranquillisers and had not felt herself for a few years. I said 'I think you have difficulty in coping with deaths'. She thought for a minute and agreed. Part of the difficulty was because both losses were very close. She was beginning to show insight and certainly wished to work through her difficulties so it was agreed between us that we should meet.

She said she had sexual difficulties within her marriage. She had been treated with dilators by a gynaecologist; she had been told that the problem was simple and would be easily cured but it had not been easy and was still with her. The 50-minute sessions took place at two-weekly intervals. In the next session she looked tense. She had noticed herself repeatedly looking at a family photograph taken when she was six years old. Her mother looked extremely ill. She then sat very quiet and began hugging herself. Coming across from her were feelings of intense sadness and misery. I felt sad, miserable, and my stomach started churning. She began discussing her feelings for her husband. He frequently came in late from work without informing her, etc. Then she talked about her enjoyment of gardening. I suggested she had difficulty in coping with her feelings of anger and hurt towards

215

her husband. She agreed but felt he could not have much happiness with her. She had not given him a child, she was not very much fun, intelligent, etc. I said 'You're putting yourself down very effectively. How could anybody like you?'. She agreed.

At the next session, she was smiling. She had had a very nice holiday with her husband, been happier than she had been for a long time. She said 'I can't bring anything miserable out of myself. You will have to throw something at me to get me going'. She went on about her holiday and then became quiet. I felt some of her guilt about enjoying talking to me about something she enjoyed. I put this to her and she agreed, saying 'I feel I'm wasting your time if I talk to you about the things I enjoy'. She immediately returned to the fact that she was terrified of the pain in labour. She was not sure whether she would breastfeed or not. Her mother had been too ill to breastfeed her. She was becoming again acutely aware of her guilt towards her mother so I stated, 'You feel there is something damaging about you. You would damage your husband if you said what you wished, you also feel you killed your mother'. To my surprise she quickly agreed: 'I feel somehow if I wasn't here my mother would be around to talk to me'. I further added 'You feel so guilty you aren't able to enjoy yourself. How could you have a happy marriage and enjoy having a baby?'

Through the next two sessions she was intensely working through her feelings of guilt. On the one hand I wished these not to be too powerful for her but on the other hand I didn't wish to protect her. Later I added 'These feelings of guilt are crippling and paralysing you'. She revealed her feelings of inadequacy, desire to escape and to perform. I said 'There is a need in you to perform. You find it difficult to be yourself'. Again there was a long period of silence, and then I added 'In the past you have coped with this feeling by retreating but now you don't know what to do with it. It's hard for you'. She replied 'No I'm not used to doing it this way'. Pointing out the ways she was reacting to me helped her to understand her own distorted reactions.

In the next session she appeared to be happy and relaxed. They had gone on another holiday. She could not remember a happier period for a long time; she had been a day late for a period. For the first time in her life she felt excited at the possibility of being pregnant, but still a little apprehensive. There was less anxiety before coming to see me. I felt there had been a very significant breakthrough but she was still a little frightened that things might go wrong. She wished for the infertility investigations to be undertaken so I went ahead with the programme. Intercourse was now enjoyable. A further session was arranged and she felt happy; but again she felt she should be pouring out her miseries but just could not do so. When I pointed out she was having some difficulty in enjoying herself she readily agreed and began laughing at herself. She then added 'When I become pregnant I wonder who will look after me?' I agreed that when she became pregnant I would look after her.

This case clearly demonstrates an emotional problem within a sub-fertile couple. There are many emotional problems resulting from the absence of a pregnancy but very clearly this patient's delayed pregnancy and even her marriage were the result of emotional problems. I have the clinical impression that a significant number of older couples who wait a long time before embarking on a family have some emotional problem. This patient was unusual in that she was able in the routine gynaecological clinic to mention these problems. I feel it would have been disastrous to have embarked on a pregnancy with such an intense feeling of guilt, but on the other hand I did not wish to delay investigations for infertility for too long — she was 35. I felt she would ask for them when she wanted them and so she did. She will probably need further help during her pregnancy.

37

The advantages of seminar training in a genetic counselling clinic

Elspeth Williamson

Genetic counselling involves estimating the risk of recurrence of specific abnormality or disease causing mental or physical handicap in a particular individual and imparting this information and its significance to the enquirer. Commonly, of course, the enquirers are a couple who are already parents or potential parents and their concern is for affected offspring. This type of clinic involves two quite distinct disciplines, first the exact biological and mathematical science of genetics, and second the less exact humanity or skill of counselling. I shall discuss only counselling and the way in which seminar training has been appropriate to it.

Most parents enquiring about risks to their offspring have become concerned about possible added risks either by a pregnancy disaster which may be a spontaneous abortion, a perinatal death, the birth of a baby with a congenital abnormality; or a childhood disaster, by which one means the birth of a baby who appears absolutely normal, but who later develops signs of either mental handicap or physical disease. This may, or may not, be of genetic origin, but most parents ask the same questions: Why did it happen? Why did it happen to me? Would it happen again?

The best way in which I can demonstrate how I have found the seminar training of use to me in genetic counselling is by giving some illustrative case histories.

Case Studies

Family A.

The first couple were referred after their first baby had been born with anencephaly. They came to see me about six months after the birth. He was a naval helicopter pilot, and she had been in the WRNS. The first remark the wife made was: 'I have had an anencephalic', not 'I have had a baby', not 'I have lost a baby', but just 'I have had' — a quite impersonal thing — 'an anencephalic'. She told me of her great tension during labour. Her husband was not able to be present, and she felt the tension mounting and when the baby was delivered, she realised that there was none of the usual excitement. She had not seen the baby but had just been told that it was an anencephalic; and the abnormality was not actually described to her. The father said he had not been allowed to see the baby either. I asked them what they thought the baby looked like. She told me that a medical directory told her that an anencephalic was a monster and that a nurse had told her that the baby had a head the size of a thumb.

They were both horrified by their own fantasies of the abnormality. When I asked them about their present sexual activity, she said 'We have not had any sex since the baby. How could I when I have had something like that inside me?'

I felt their sense of sexual failure in having the abnormal baby, her sense of inadequacy and horror that she had produced a monster, the terrible fantasy that they both had built up about it. When I mentioned that the child had arms and legs and other normal structures, they hardly believed me. They had been referred to me so that I could give them the risks of recurrence of this particular abnormality. They wanted to know this, of course, but the help they really needed was the help we give to patients with psychosexual problems. Her cry was 'I am not normal'.

I think this couple does raise one problem. Should they have seen the baby at birth, and come to terms with the severe abnormality? Should a socially acceptable photograph of the baby dressed in clothes, and the abnormality hidden as best as possible by a bonnet been shown to them, or should we have left them just as they were? Let us look again at the two questions: Why dit it happen? Why did it happen to me?

When answering these questions in diseases and abnormalities due to single genes, we are saying 'This is genetic in origin and you passed an abnormal gene on to your child'. So we are, in this situation, assigning guilt to one or other parent.

The next family I will describe to you perhaps illustrates the tremendous aggression and guilt feelings that this assignment of responsibility can raise within families.

Family B.

A child had been born suffering from tuberosclerosis and was severely retarded. The condition is due to a single autosomal gene of major effect, which shows its effect in single dose, and therefore, if one or other parent carries this gene, there is a one-in-two risk that he will pass it on to any of his offspring. As in so many of the dominant conditions, the same gene can produce very varying effects in different individuals carrying it, some much milder than others. In this family the father was found to have the shagreen patch and some small de-pigmented areas of an aspen leaf shape, indicating that he was, in fact, carrying this gene and it was he who had passed it on to the severely retarded child. The risk of it happening again was one chance in two.

The couple came into my consulting room, first the wife, very positive, very aggressive, very cross, bringing with her the first and normal child, then the father, with the retarded child. He slunk into the room and sat in the corner, rather hunched up. The wife then produced her ideas about having more children which she desperately wanted. She was cross with everybody because of what had happened and she assigned all the guilt to her husband, who sat by meekly and accepted it all. Of course, they realised that it would be unwise to have another child because of the high risk of further abnormality, but the wife was using the tool of wanting another child to vent aggression upon her unfortunate husband. One felt that this family needed help in coming to terms with what had happened to them, perhaps as a couple, not purely as single individuals.

Family C.

Another case where there was tremendous aggression, was a girl who suffered from Von Hippel Lindau disease and was partially sighted. She was married to a diabetic who was sub-fertile and she had come asking for artificial insemination. When I told her that Von Hippel Lindau disease was an autosomal dominant condition, and that one in two of her children would suffer from it, maybe more severely than herself so that I did not feel that artificial insemination was indicated, she rose up from her chair in her wrath, threw a mass of vituperation at me and walked out of the door, slamming it behind her harder than I have ever heard anybody slam the door. However she did send me a Christmas card that year and said that really she quite agreed with me and she hoped she was coming to terms with the situation.

The other genetic conditions one sees which are carried by single genes are only manifest when present in double dose, the so-called recessive conditions. These genes are carried in single dose by absolutely normal people and in fact each of us carries six or seven of these recessive genes, but most of us do not know what we are carrying. Unfortunately, when an affected child is born with a recessive condition, then both parents are identified as being carriers of the recessive gene.

Family D.

> One family I saw who had a child with cystic fibrosis came to see me about the risk of recurrence. I told them that both of them must be carriers of this condition, and that there was a one-in-four risk of recurrence in future children. They were both quite shattered and overcome by their own guilt. They said they felt like lepers. This particular couple did not have a very stable marriage, both were somewhat inadequate people and yet, because of their guilt feelings and their inability to cope, they were somehow colluding to hold together a most unhealthy relationship. Their sexual life had been very limited and in no way satisfying, certainly for the wife.

In x-linked diseases, which only affect males and are carried by absolutely normal females, one again has this very difficult task of assigning guilt to one of a partnership. I have often encountered aggression because a mother has given birth to an affected boy and I have had to tell her not only that it was her fault that the child was affected but also that she carries a risk of a further affected boy.

Another group one sees referred to a genetic counselling clinic are what we might call the poor reproducers. These are families which have recurrent pregnancy failures which seem unrelated, perhaps an abortion or a still birth followed by a child with some form of congenital abnormality. Rarely do we find a genetic cause for these, but of course the distress to the family and their sense of failure is very marked.

The counsellor must try to help these parents through their feelings of inadequacy because of this failure which has been experienced by other people within the family.

Finally, I would look at the question of why patients come when they do come. I have had patients who have taken as long as eight years between the referral letter and coming to see me. I think patients come to genetic counselling clinics at a time of crisis following some form of disaster. When it is eight years later, one should wonder what crisis has just happened and one can suspect often and perhaps confirm that this is a marital crisis.

What is genetic counselling all about? Is it a purely genetic situation, in which one is saying the condition that damaged your baby is genetic, or is not genetic, and this is the risk of recurrence? To what extent should we be interpreting the significance of the risk? We can explain that if the baby with the condition is going to be born dead, then the risk is purely a risk to the parents of suffering the tragedy of a second death, whereas if the child is going to be severely handicapped and may survive ten or 15 years with a deteriorating condition, then this risk involves not only the parents, but the child as well, and possibly the other siblings. Should I just bury my Institute-trained head in the sand and not listen to the undertones of distress that come across? I think I can only end by saying that in my view it is quite useless to reassure the patients if you have not understood their needs.

Part IX Sexual abuse

This section concludes with two papers on the, hopefully, more infrequent situations: counselling women who have suffered rape and counselling patients in HM prisons.

38

Reactions to rape

Judy Gilley

In this presentation I shall hope to cover four aspects of this difficult and topical subject. First, my involvement in the treatment of women who have been raped; second 'Who sees women who have been raped?'; third, research on responses to rape; and fourth, a case study.

My personal involvement
This originated whilst I was working in a neighbourhood health centre in Indiana, USA, in 1973. I was surprised by the numbers of women who came quietly to request a gynaecological examination — 'to be sure everything is OK'. In the process of the vaginal examination they would reveal, often with distress, that they had been raped. These were mainly 'minority group women'. Many appeared not to have reported the attack to anyone.

There were at that time particularly horrific rapes in the city where I worked, involving both very young girls and elderly women. This led to increased public concern and ultimately the formation of a Rape Crisis Centre, largely organised by feminist groups. I was medical adviser to the centre and met many women who had been raped in the past or recently.

On returning to this country I spoke about 'the American experience', questioning whether we had a similar hidden problem in this country. I was greeted with incredulity, and horror, especially in medical circles. In July 1974 I wrote an article for *New Society* 'How to help the raped' (Gilley 1974). This precipitated an enormous correspondence from women all over the country who wanted help or wanted to help others who had been raped. During the years 1975–76 a group of concerned women, mainly feminists, with a variety of skills, worked to establish the first Rape Crisis Centre here, which is now flourishing in London. I was proud to work with them.

Who sees women who have been raped?
Whilst police surgeons are involved at the time of reporting of a rape, they do not usually play a part in the continuing physical and mental care of the woman. Family doctors may be aware of one or two cases of rape within their practice, especially if a young girl is involved and is brought by her parents. Psychiatrists

appear to see few women who have been raped. Family planning doctors, especially those with psychosexual training, may be aware of women with sexual problems following rape, and frequently these may not present until some years after the event.

The majority of women in the London area who are raped are seen by women workers at the Rape Crisis Centre. The formation of such centres has been described in detail elsewhere (Gilley 1974). In the first 18 months of its establishment the Rape Crisis Centre had some 322 direct contacts with women who had been raped and 71 women had been referred to them by other agencies (Rape Crisis Centre 1978, 1979). The centre is run by volunteers who are trained especially to help raped women, many of whom find it easier to relate to a 'non-professional' woman who can empathise with their ordeal. Obviously such centres must have ready access to medical and legal advice, and good connections with local VD clinics, gynaecologists, psychiatrists and family planning clinics. They must be able to recognise that the needs of some women demand more specialised help than they can offer.

Many women report rape only long after the event (perhaps years later) when their psychological needs are pressing. The legal and other niceties which so frighten us doctors have long since become irrelevant. Legal aspects of rape have been described elsewhere (Gilley 1980). I feel that it is at this later stage that doctors trained by the Institute have valuable skills to offer a woman who presents for help.

Responses to rape
Research to date comes almost entirely from the USA. No funding has yet been made available for research here. I will summarise the most significant research.

Burgess & Holmstrong (1974) largely confirm the earlier findings of Sutherland & Scherl (1970). These workers followed 92 adult women for one year after they had been raped. This was a heterogenous sample, age range 17 to 73, of normal cultural and class distribution. They identified three stages in what they described as the Rape Trauma Syndrome:

1. An acute phase in which there is much disorganisation of life-style, in which physical symptoms predominate and in which anxiety and fear are prevalent. The physical symptoms include:
    a. Those relating to the physical trauma experienced.
    b. Skeletal muscle tension, sleep pattern disturbances — crying out in the sleep.
    c. Gastro-intestinal irritability — abdominal pains, anorexia, nausea.
    d. Genito-urinary symptoms — vaginal discharge, cystitis and generalised pelvic pain.
    e. Rectal bleeding where there has been anal sex.

2. In the second phase the woman begins to reorganise her life-style — perhaps two to three weeks after the attack. She may move or go abroad; she may turn to her family for support; she may develop fear of indoors or outdoors according to the site of the rape; she may be fearful of being alone or in

223

crowds. Sexual fears surface, which may be especially upsetting if there has been no previous sexual experience, or resumption of pre-existing sexual relationships may be severely affected. During this second stage the woman may appear outwardly to have adjusted well, usually returning to work or school, but there is a heavy measure of denial expressed in such phrases as 'It could have happened to anyone'. Little interest is shown in gaining insight.

3. In phase three or 'resolution' the majority of women become depressed and need to talk. Anxieties, already dealt with superficially, reappear. This phase involves acceptance of the event and the woman must resolve her feelings of anger, etc. about the assailant. This stage may be precipitated by a court appearance, which is often a great ordeal for the woman, especially if the man is not convicted or is given a suspended sentence. This may rekindle fear of another attack, and many women feel they have been proven 'guilty' by a non-conviction.

I would also like to mention the work of Sharon McCombie (1975). In 1975 she did a one-year follow-up of 70 women who had been raped. Her main preoccupation was with the relationship between the behaviour of the woman at the time of the rape and her subsequent feelings about the way she handled the rape: 35 per cent of the women in her study had offered no resistance; 19 per cent had screamed and 11 per cent had used physical force to resist. Those who had not resisted were plagued with thoughts that they could have avoided rape if they had struggled. In all, 18 per cent were seriously troubled by their role in the attack. McCombie related this anxiety about role to the developmental stage of these women. Many were young women beginning to separate from their families, hoping to establish their independence, and exploring their sexuality. The rape appeared to rob them of their autonomy and precipitated major concerns about their competency to function as independent individuals.

Case Study

In this study I have attempted to highlight the reactions of an individual woman to being raped. There is therefore relatively little concentration on therapeutic technique and 'interventions'.

This concerns Grace, a young woman of 22. She was referred initially by her GP to whom her mother had taken her when it was discovered that she had been raped. On the first occasion I saw her she came alone. She had been raped two weeks previously. She was thin, pale, fair, nervous and near to tears. I said I was very glad that she had come and asked her gently how she was. She replied between sobs 'Physically I'm OK, but I've got a heavy vaginal discharge which makes me feel sick. I was given some pessaries a week ago and I've been to a VD clinic and have to go back. I feel sick and angry. I want to do something about it'.

J.A.G.	Do you mean prosecute?
GRACE	Yes, I suppose so.
J.A.G.	Have you reported the rape to the police?
GRACE	No, It's too late. I can't.
J.A.G.	Does anyone know?
GRACE	My parents: it was obvious to them from the state I was in when I got home, and some friends at work, I think. [*Tears.*]

224

J.A.G.   Would you like to talk about what happened?

[With great difficulty, often with tears, sometimes missing bits out and going back, she described the rape. In order to preserve her confidentiality, I will not describe the details leading to the rape. In summary she was raped by a minicab driver. There have been a spate of such rapes in London involving minicabs recently.]

GRACE   Originally I wasn't too worried. He tried to persuade me to go back to his place. I refused. Then he refused to take me any further and stopped the car. He said he would phone another cab to take me home. It was late and cold and I was getting worried. He invited me in whilst he phoned and I was worried but I would have felt a bit of a fool standing on the pavement at 1 a.m. so I went in. Once we got into that room, something happened. He looked at me and I felt very frightened. He hit me and started to shout at me. I was terrified. He said he would kill me and started to tear at my clothes. I was screaming, but when I screamed he hit me more so I started asking why he was doing it. He threw me to the gound and said 'Don't try any of that stuff on me, don't try to understand me. I hate women'. He raped me. It hurt a lot. I cried. I was shivering. He went into the next room and then he came back. I thought Oh God, this is it. But he threw me out into the street with a bundle of clothes. I can't remember much about getting home. I got a taxi in the end. Crying all the time and my father heard me when I got back. I feel I want to get back at him.
J.A.G.   What were you thinking of?
GRACE   I don't know what I can do. I'm not sleeping, not eating. I'm having bad dreams. I feel anxious about all men. I even feel angry with my father. [*Tears.*] I'm worried about getting pregnant.
J.A.G.   Where were you in your cycle?
GRACE   Near the beginning, I think, but if my period doesn't come I won't be able to stand it. I can't wait for a pregnancy test. [*Tears.*]

It emerged that she had been on the pill for a steady relationship until six months previously and that she had been at approximately day eight of a cycle when attacked.

The interview ended with details of how she could contact me and of her VD appointment for the continuing vaginal discharge. In summary it seemed this first interview was a time for her to feel able to speak, for careful listening. I felt she needed to know that I was sympathetic, understood something of the ordeal she had been through, and would help. It was not a time for interpretations, and it was not possible to follow through any one issue; her thoughts were flitting from one anxiety to the next. Two days later she phoned because there was a minicab outside her house. She was in a state of total panic. I talked to her for several minutes on the phone until the cab drew away and she was able to relax. I said I was glad that she had felt able to phone me. For myself I felt glad that I had been easily available to establish that I would help whenever I could.

At the second interview, some four days after the first, she was somewhat less distressed initially, but then intermittently very tearful because gonorrhoea had been confirmed by the special clinic.

GRACE   I feel filthy. [*Weeping.*] I feel contaminated. I hate my body like this. I've seen my boy friend. [A steady relationship of several years.] I told him but it was very difficult. He says he understands how I feel but he doesn't know how much I'm repulsed by the idea of him touching me *at all.*

The third interview took place some 11 days after the first. Grace was still weeping, she looked pale and ill and thin. Intermittently she was very angry. She said 'I'm considering going to the police'.

We discussed once again the technical possibilities of reporting and the possibilities for successful prosecution at this stage. We talked about what it would mean for her. I asked her what she was hoping for from a prosecution. She replied 'Revenge'.

This was said with great emphasis. The thought of pregnancy was also occupying her — her period was now three days late. 'I can't have a test. I couldn't bear to know if it was positive.'

We talked about the possibility of a menstrual extraction should a test be positive. Together we decided to wait for a few more days.

By the end of this interview my anxieties for her were growing, particularly because of the weight loss, and her continued anorexia. I felt the need to produce a miracle for her which was what she wanted for herself.

There followed a great number of phone calls to organise an 'early' pregnancy test and finally a conversation with a sympathetic gynaecologist who understood her needs and said 'You're asking me to do a Ritual Cleansing for her'. At the end of the following week this was done. Grace wanted only to hear that there was now no way she could be pregnant. Later she sent me a thank-you note.

The fourth interview was some six weeks after the rape. She expressed her relief at the menstrual extraction, although she had found it painful and grim. However, now she developed another vaginal discharge. 'Won't this ever end? My body won't let me forget. I do occasionally forget in fact. I'm thinking of leaving my job.'

She now weighed six stone. Because of her increasing anorexia and depression, her GP had just started her on Ludiomil.

The fifth interview was the next day. She came back unexpectedly. She had not taken any Ludiomil. Immediately she started the conversation by saying that she wanted to talk about her father.

GRACE   I don't feel he cares. I want something from him.
J.A.G.   How are things between you?
GRACE   We used to be very close. I get on better with him than my mother. My parents are arguing a lot since this happened. I think he's ashamed of me. I think his job and reputation mean more to him than I do. [*Tears.*]
J.A.G.   What would you have wanted him to do?
GRACE   Beat him [the rapist] up. Get the police. [*Her voice tailed off.*] I don't know. [*An air of resignation and despair.*]
J.A.G.   He must be feeling very useless, very frustrated, very guilty.
GRACE   I suppose so, but I can't feel the same about him. I can't bear to touch him. We used to be so close.
J.A.G.   That must be so painful for you when you've been so close. [*She then wept for a long time and we shared her pain.*]

The sixth interview took place two months after the rape. She had returned to work and at least her bodily symptoms were beginning to settle. We were both relieved. The seventh interview was three months after the rape. Again she came unexpectedly to the surgery. She was very upset, she had been back to the VD clinic for a routine check and had seen another doctor. He told her there was some pus on the cervix and had given her some tablets. She was very afraid that this might be gonorrhoea again come back to haunt her. 'Shall I check it for you?' 'Yes please.'

I knew this was very important to her. She wanted more than a clean bill of health. She got on to the couch, holding one hand over her face which was contorted. She remained silent throughout. There was no vaginismus. It was an easy examination and the cervix was perfectly clean. I told her 'It looks very good to me. Everything feels good and healthy'. She relaxed a little, but I felt she was still distancing herself from the vaginal examination.

J.A.G.   How do you feel? [*Silence only.*] Have you made love with your boy friend?
GRACE   Not *yet*. I don't want to. [*She sat up.*] Thank you anyway.

There was a slight smile as she got up and a general air of relief. I phoned the venereologist. There had been nothing specific on the examination; he had given her the oxytetracycline 'as a precaution'. I told her this and she was very relieved.

The eighth interview was four months after the rape. She had gained weight. She was much more bouncy. There were some smiles. She had given up her job and decided to travel. She described it as an extended holiday. The relationship with her boy friend had ended. However, she had gone back on the pill.

J.A.G.	That can't be bad. [*She smiled.*]
GRACE	I wanted to show you the book I've been reading about rape [*Medea & Thompson, 1974.*]. I've underlined bits that seemed important to me, things that make sense to me: 'Rape is a violation of a woman's sexual determination' and a longer one 'Whenever a woman walks alone at night, enters a pub, hitchhikes, she is aware that she is violating well-established rules of conduct, and as a result that she faces the possibility of rape. If in one of these situations she is raped, the man will almost certainly escape prosecution and the woman will be made to feel responsible because she was somehow asking for it.'
J.A.G.	I know the book, I can understand the difficulty and the pain in what you've underlined.

I think this was the nearest she could come to expressing the guilt she felt about being raped. She was preoccupied with her behaviour at the time — for example, having entered his room — and this raised considerable problems for her for the future: 'How will I handle similar situations in the future?'

One year later Grace was still abroad.

39

Counselling in HM prisons

Patricia Roberts

Some years ago I was given the opportunity to work with psychosexual problems in our local men's prison. It was an experimental project initially for six months and no one was certain what the response or outcome would be. It seemed likely that most sexual offenders would be labelled psychopathic and therefore outside the scope of our seminar training, and in prison any heterosexual counselling must be largely hypothetical. However, even in a prison with a caring reputation such as this one, no therapy would be offered without an overt request or recommendation and many completed their sentence without ever discussing their offence or their feelings about it.

There were already two medical officers with psychiatric qualifications, another male member of the Institute and a visiting consultant psychiatrist on the staff. The hospital's officers particularly feared that the men might think this a soft option and the enterprise was doomed to failure.

Perhaps my first patient was a test case — he could have been intended to discourage me. He was a wiry, voluble little man with a Midlands accent, speech impediment and missing front teeth, demanding to see a sexologist. For 20 minutes he raged about the prison system before telling me with some diffidence (and after enquiring first as to whether I were a married lady) that he had a 'small penis'. I thought we built up a reasonable rapport, but after the second visit he went back and bashed up his cell. As this is one of the few means of venting frustration in prison, no one was too dismayed, but when after the third session he emptied his chamber pot over an officer's head, disciplinary action was swift. Everyone was politely reassuring — he would probably have done it anyway without my help — but it was not an auspicious beginning. The case was, in fact, quite harrowing. Serving a life sentence for a murder that was almost accidental, he had been in prison just too long. Each time parole was pending, the anxiety became so unbearable that he reacted with violence. Unfortunately, he was moved to another prison almost immediately and I did not see him again.

Further referrals included two men who had stabbed their wives, a rapist lorry-driver and an incestuous father: domestic situations where it was just possible to speculate whether an earlier visit to a marital problems session might have prevented tragedy.

Had the wife agreed to have her prolapse repaired and the husband's anxiety over damaging her been ventilated, would he have been driven to stab her with his screw-driver? If the second wife had sought help for her frigidity, would this miserable little man now be serving five years for seeking comfort from his daughter? Had the lorry-driver not categorised his women so rigidly into Madonnas and whores, need he have tied his woman naked to a tree in the park with her clothes neatly folded just out of reach? These were obviously over-simplifications but suggested that there might be scope for working along accustomed lines. Everything here seemed a little larger than life. These were men who had acted out their fantasies or whose fantasies had taken over.

Although these men seeking help may not have been completely truthful concerning their offences, they were devastatingly honest about their present feelings. As in a crisis situation, very little intervention produced surprising results; and precepts and truths sought diligently in the seminar became readily recognisable. It was as though, in this state of isolation from the outside world, stripped of their clothing as it were, they were more ready to bare their souls also.

My first patient complained of a small penis and, when the second and third also did, I took this to be interesting evidence of regression, until it occurred to me that this had something to do with the doctors' difficulty in regarding these men as other than naughty little boys.

Apart from loss of freedom and loss of family life, perhaps with breakdown of marriage, a sexual offender suffers loss of respect and self-esteem, which was probably never very high at the best of times. He is at the bottom of the prison social scale. If the offence involved children, he frequently has to be segregated for his personal safety.

Punishment, in this instance, imprisonment, is important to most offenders, who wish to pay back their debt to society. By a minority, it may be seen as a much-needed if adverse form of attention, but others have a need to atone for acts of which they are ashamed. Their horror at what they have done, or at the strength of the emotions they have been unable to control, is often so great that they develop a partial or total amnesia for the sequence of events. It was exciting to find that by using our techniques to reach pain and fantasy, the amnesia might be lifted. This was desirable if we were to discuss the fear of repetition.

N.'s pain was reached through the shame of a negative sperm count (a fact he had never admitted), which had almost driven him to castrate a homosexual youth. The result of the count had been sent through the post on Christmas Eve and led to the breakdown of his marriage.

John, who had rammed a piece of wood down a woman's throat, was suddenly able to recall the details on the eve of his own tonsillectomy. While discussing his apprehension over the operation, he talked of his mother's hysterectomy ('they left *bits* behind') revealing terrifying fantasies of damaging her during his birth, recurrent nightmares of being pushed violently through a long tunnel. This boy needed a lot of support, growing up rapidly in the first year he spent in an adult prison. Eagerly, he talked through his childhood sexual feelings towards his mother. He loved her so much he wanted 'to get in bed with her'.

Denial and repression had been Tom's pattern of coping with pain and loss all through life, his offence coming as a climax after repeated loss situations and rejections imperfectly worked through. A classic separation anxiety in a children's hospital, social deprivation and fortuitous calamity left him unable to cope with the normal pattern of attachment and loss to communicate sexually with his wife. The explosion, when it came, was bizarre and apparently unrelated to the casual frustration which was relatively minor. He sank two bottles of Spanish wine at his mother's house, ran home, poured paraffin over the dog, set it alight and stabbed his wife in the stomach when she came to its rescue, then ran amok holding off a posse of police.

He presented shaking from head to foot, mumbling incomprehensibly, occasionally managing a short phrase. His wife felt she must leave him unless the doctor could assure her that he would not do this again. We worked back through the long history of rejections, both real and imaginary and had a very valuable joint interview in which his anxiety at her late arrival was revealing. They talked over their difficulties in communication and now keep very closely in touch over everything. He survived refusal of parole very well, thinking first of the disappointment for his wife, and he has matured in a remarkable way.

However, not everyone presents with gloom and despondency. There are characters like Flash Harry to brighten the scene. Harry was referred with some apologies — 'I wonder if you would see him — not a marital problem — but a compulsive gambler whose wife keeps writing to get help for him'.

Harry is an engaging character. His shirt is well laundered and starched (he knows how to arrange these things) and he wears tinted spectacles, legitimately as it happens, for recurrent iritis. He knows too, how to handle women, leaning nonchalantly across the desk to flick his ash into the waste paper basket by my side, withdrawing his hand quickly I notice, like a little boy expecting a smack on the wrist. His colourful language and vivid turn of phrase would provide years of after-dinner anecdotes for carefully selected audiences.

His first three marriages had ended in disaster and he was now living with the common-law wife who showed such concern. His comments on this were memorable: 'Me a marriage problem? Don't you get me wrong doctor. I'm a faithful man. While I'm married I keep my cock indoors.'

Harry has lived on his wits all his life. At 40, he is still unable to read or write. Skilled at his job, he has depended on his good wives to balance his accounts and place his bets. Each in turn thought she would change him and enjoyed his little-boy charm until the restrictions began to irk and bore him. He developed a need to denigrate and humiliate his women. Craving a high level of excitement, he would gamble away the lot. He is anxious to change — 'You gotta help me doc!' — but he needs room to manoeuvre and has now gone off on a painting and decorating course. He says he needs to come back and I find I am anxious to see him. It is debatable how long I too will last.

Homosexuality

I am frequently asked about homosexuality. There is of course much homosexuality in prison. The revelation for me has been the infinite range of reactions and attitudes towards it. Men are forced in a unique way to consider their total sexuality. As one young man put it: 'I have come to the conclusion that I am 60 per cent male and 30 per cent female — do you think that a fair assessment?' We never quite decided about the other 10 per cent.

Some seem to have settled for masturbation with heterosexual fantasy. Those with doubts over their masculinity are more threatened and confused. From one of these I had a run down on the prison sexual hierarchy, ranging from heterosexual 'wolves' who demand homosexual submission to the 'faggots' who offer themselves passively — all this while he tried to find his own level on the scale.

One confirmed homosexual I have as a patient, fell as a crumb from the psychiatrist's table. A charming, personable, slightly narcissistic young man who does not seek help for his homosexuality, but for his attraction to adolescent youths — one in particular.

Were it not for the discipline of seminar training, I should have been wildly searching for clues as to the reason for his homosexuality. Instead I find I can tolerate the anxieties — which he introduces each time as 'amusing' but ending with the phrase 'I do find this disturbing'.

The doctor-patient relationship
The knowledge that the doctor may have to write a report for the parole board or prison of next referral can interfere with the doctor-patient relationship. On the whole, we are both aware this is happening and I did think I had developed a technique for dealing with this hazard. On at least two occasions, however, additional information (mainly factual) has been produced after the parole result was known — once in gratitude for a positive outcome and once in the pain and anger of a parole refusal, just to show me I wasn't as clever as I thought.

I personally find reports difficult. There are facts to bog you down. Who is going to read them? There is at least one psychiatrist on the parole board, but also departments where the mention of fantasy can render a man suspect. I never include anything confidential or, if possible, anything adverse unless it can be affirmed that, with insight, the man may be or has already changed.

Frequently, I am right out of my depth and utterly dependent on what I have retained from seminar training. Without it, I would regularly be anxious as to what I should *do* and take flight into action, rather than sit it out and wait for what the patient will offer.

This is particularly true with the persistent sexual offender. What can one *do* with a man like Jim charged with buggery 72 times? Jim decided this for himself. He asked to discuss his sexual development.

In general, the difficulty lies in forming any adult relationship at all. Few have the ability to chat up a girl and segregation, of course, does nothing to develop social skills. None of my present small group of child molesters have shown any violence, none have gained much pleasure from their actions and none have sought adult homosexual relationships. Their sexual inferiority appears total.

I do try to keep a focus in mind, but it may have to be broadly based. In this situation one has to be prepared to play many different roles, without being too proud and purist about it; anything from witch to wet-nurse, social adviser, bereavement counsellor or safe confidante. (Frequently, I hear of minor undetected crimes like readdressing parcels to yourself when working with British Rail.)

231

Timing has to be geared to the needs of a man who may have no idea when he will be released.

Conclusions
The results of evaluating my work in prison are not very startling:

1. A small number of prisoners, depressed and fearful over their sexuality, can now accept it and if they get out in time may even enjoy it.
2. A few have shown remarkable personal growth. The opportunity to share their load of guilt and anxiety in a safe setting, to be accepted 'warts and all' has enabled them to regain some self-respect.
3. I believe a number are unlikely to offend again in the same way.
4. More men are asking for help and we sometimes have a waiting list.

Some wise person said that as long as we feel our participation is worthwhile, we shall find ourselves able to tolerate high levels of disturbance in others without disengaging. I have no doubt that it is worthwhile. Between the frankly psychopathic and the border-line ESN, there is a grey area where vulnerable, inadequate and lonely men display behaviour differing only in degree from many who turn up in clinics and surgeries. Prison does not seem to be the place for them after the initial period of atonement.

It may be my fantasy that our sort of participation can do much to rehabilitate and return them usefully and with some hope of joy to the community. Far too many have been shut out and conveniently forgotten.

One prison governor I know read to a prison assembly from 'The Dry Salvages' a passage which is true for all our patients and also for ourselves, but particularly applicable to the sort of men I have just described, those who are shut out and in a state of transition.

> Fare forward, you who think you are voyaging;
> You are not those who saw the harbour
> Receding, or those who will disembark,
> Here between the hither and the farther shore
> While time is withdrawn, consider the future
> And the past with an equal mind.

Hopefully, at what T. S. Eliot calls 'The moment which is not of action or inaction', the doctor-patient relationship will work its strange alchemy.

Appendices

Appendix I contains the programme of the Conference. As well as invited papers, there were a number of Free Communications. Speakers who gave Free Communications were asked to submit an abstract; for those who failed to supply one I have included the summary from their original submission. Appendix I also includes an abbreviated text of the Director of Training's remarks on the design of the Conference and her summing up of the meeting which, with the President's closing address, reiterate not only the themes of the Conference but also the ideas that have been explored in this book.

Appendix II gives the provenance of the papers other than those given at the Conference.

Appendix III provides information about the Institute of Psychosexual Medicine, including the regulations for training, membership and accreditation.

Appendix I

Programme of the First International Conference on Psychosexual
Medicine held at the Brighton Metropole Hotel, 7-10 July, 1982

Wednesday 7 July. Session 1
The design of the conference   *Dr P. Tunnadine*
Training for acquisition of knowledge or development of skill? (Introductory
address)   *Dr T. Main*

Thursday 8 July. Session 2 (Chairman: *Dr Barbara Law*)
Covert presentation of psychosexual problems   *Dr R. Freedman*
Youth advisory work   *Dr F. Hutchinson*

Session 3 (Chairman: *Miss Valerie Thompson*)
Non-consummation   *Dr M. Bramley*
Retarded ejaculation   *Dr R. Lincoln and Dr R. Thexton*

FREE COMMUNICATIONS (Chairman: *Dr T. Main*)
Analysis of referrals to a psychosexual clinic in a psychiatric setting in an attempt to
conduct a follow-up study   *Dr S. Proctor*
Genital pain in men   *Dr D. MacDonald Burns*
Sexuality and body image   *Dr E. Koadlow*
Extracts from film *Breaking the Ice*   *Dr A. Begg*

Friday 9 July. Session 4 (Chairman: *Dr Joan Marshall*)
Secondary frigidity (postnatal loss of libido)   *Dr A. Tobert*
Impotence   *Dr J. Berry and Dr J. Yorston*

Session 5 (Chairman: *Mrs Nancy Raphael*)
Exploration of the dynamics of seeing couples   *Dr K. Draper*
Problems presenting in contraceptive work   *Dr. E. Christopher*

FREE COMMUNICATIONS (Chairman: *Dr T. Main*)
Emotional problems associated with infertile patients   *Dr F. Johnson*
Climacterium: a psychochological perspective   *Dr K. Chinoy*
Dependence and independence   *Dr J. Kilvington*
Follow-up research in vaginismus   *Prof. H. Musaph*
The risks of oral and anal intercourse   *Dr J. Black*

Saturday 10 July. Session 6 (Chairman: *Dr Elsie Koadlow*)
Requests for termination of pregnancy   *Dr M. Blair*
   (read by Dr J. Pasmore)
Sterilisation (Personal recollections of the vasectomy research seminar)
Dr P. Tunnadine

Session 7
Director of Training's concluding remarks   *Dr P. Tunnadine*
President's closing address   *Dr T. Main*

The design of the Conference

Prudence Tunnadine

My name is Pru Tunnadine. Like the rest of you, I am a doctor who meets, in the course of her everyday work, patients who find their love-life disappointing and who seek my help to improve it.

Having looked at your preliminary programme you will realise that we have invited you here to take part in a funny kind of Conference — one that is inventive and experimental, perhaps unique, but certainly impossible.

This task is impossible for two reasons. First of all it is clearly not feasible that in three days and a dozen short papers we can give you a detailed account of the clinical studies, training, research and development of 25 years' work.

We have not asked our speakers to attempt to give you tight scientific accounts. We have asked them just to talk about the flavour of their work, to give you the feel of the way we think about the topics, as an introduction to the group seminar discussions.

This leads to the second impossible thing: neither is it possible in concentrated work over three days really to show you how it feels to be in an Institute training seminar, because in a training seminar we meet, we discuss our case work, and then go away for a fortnight. You would chew over in your own mind, decide what was useful and what was rubbish, and you would use it or not use it with your patients; and you would then come back and report whether it had proved useful or not. This is not possible here, but we do hope that in arranging the Conference this way you will at least have the maximum opportunity to participate: to discuss your own methods of dealing with patients with an Institute leader.

Free Communications

Abstracts

Analysis of referrals to a psychosexual clinic in a psychiatric setting and an attempt to conduct a follow-up study   *S. E. Proctor*

All referrals to a psychosexual clinic held in the Department of Psychiatry in a teaching hospital over a five-year period were analysed by source of referral and presenting problem. An attempt was then made to follow up these patients to identify the important elements of treatment, particularly from the patients' point of view.

The sample of 98 men and 66 women were mostly referred by their GP (69 per cent). Other sources of referral were endocrinologists (15 per cent) and gynaecologists (9 per cent), the remainder coming from other hospital doctors or social workers.

Analysis showed that 32 per cent of these referrals presented with a sexual problem not usually included within the 'sexual dysfunctions' and this probably reflected the psychiatric setting of the clinic. Thirteen per cent had gender dysphoria problems — transexualism, transvestism or homosexuality, and 8 per cent had more widespread psychiatric disorders such as monosymptomatic psychosis (three cases) and schizophrenia (two).

The commonest presenting problem in the 'sexual dysfunction' group was secondary erectile failure which, together with the primary cases, comprised 29 per cent. The next commonest presentation was lack of or loss of desire, particularly in women (13 per cent), and the other dysfunctions were relatively few, notably three men with premature ejaculation and four couples with non-consummation.

Participation in the follow-up study was requested by letter which produced a rather disappointing response rate of 49 per cent with only 42 people (26 per cent) prepared to come for interview. The retrospective design of the study may partially explain the low rate, as may the 'psychiatric' bias of referrals, but the main reason is probably to be found in the fact that most of those who did not respond had also not completed treatment, a reflection of the sensitivity and ambivalence of this group of patients to their sexual problems.

Subjective improvement during treatment had been maintained by 16 of the 29 'dysfunctional' patients, the most important factor in their treatment being the work done on the non-sexual aspects of their relationships, particularly if they were seen with their partner. Specific sexual techniques were mostly seen as irrelevant and occasionally mentioned as the reason for defaulting from therapy. Women fared better than men and were more likely to have attended with a partner. Those referred from other hospital departments fared less well, perhaps as they were less likely to see their problems in psychological terms.

Further prospective studies are needed to identify more clearly factors leading to improvement or abandonment of therapy.

Climacterium: a psychological perspective   *K. B. Chinoy*

This paper was written after a time-limited group therapy with women in the climacteric age group. It outlines the events occurring during climacterium, their impact on a person's life, and how to manage them.

Events occurring during climacterium

Ageing is experienced in cultural context. If a culture places a high value on youth and productivity, the experience of ageing may be difficult. On the other hand, if a culture sees ageing as a process of maturity and reaping wisdom, then it may be a welcome change and accepted with good grace. Physical changes such as obesity, growth of facial hair, cessation of menstrual periods, vulnerability to physical illness, declining vision and hearing may have a negative psychological impact on the individual's self-image. Vulnerability to physical illness reminds one of one's mortality.

Menopause is accompanied by profound somatic and endocrine changes. Psychological experience of menopause is influenced by personality factors, psychosexual identity and myths about menopause. Although it may be a passing phase of discomfort in a well-adjusted woman, it can cause profound depression if a woman's feminine and psychosexual identity is threatened. Sexuality *per se* remains unchanged.

Empty nest syndrome occurs when teenage children leave home. Once the nest is empty, the parents feel depressed.

Identity crisis is experienced when parenthood comes to an end. Termination of parenthood requires defining a new identity in terms of new roles, and new careers.

Marital changes surface when children leave home. Partners may find each other total strangers, especially if they have grown apart. Separation and divorce can occur at this time.

Significant other losses occur at this phase of life. Many important figures are passing away like parents, spouses and friends. One can face isolation if one fails to reinvest in new relationships.

Psychological implications

Sadness or depression can be an obvious reaction to loss and change. Hence, mourning is an important key to the successful outcome of climacterium. If the grief and depression can be worked through, new creativity can surface. One can accomplish a new identity accompanied with serenity and maturity.

While hormone therapy can be useful to some women, it does not change attitudes or modes of experience. On the other hand, individual and group therapy is very useful. Goals in therapy would be: (1) Elimination of myths and education about facts. (2) Mourning of losses. (3) Building self-esteem. (4) Defining a new identity and a new role in society. (5) Self-realisation.

Dependence and independence   *Jane Kilvington*

It is a common observation that some people find it difficult to work in partnership. The problem is common to both men and women and seems to be a failure of balancing the need to give leadership with the willingness, in turn, to be led. In a sexual partnership the lack of this alternation of dependence and independence may cause a breakdown in the relationship. One wonders if the failure is rooted in childhood experiences.

A pleasant but restrained woman of 26 years sought help because soon after marriage she had lost all wishes for sexual intercourse and recently she had only endured it with pain. She described her first relationship at 15 years in which she escaped from her controlling father and her religious mother only to discover that her partner was very demanding, ultimately threatening suicide when she tried to withdraw. She was not only frightened but felt overwhelmingly bad that she had caused so much unhappiness.

The vaginal examination was limited by vaginismus but the doctor learnt more when the patient said she liked gentle doctors and found a brusque one upsetting. She began to talk about her wishes to keep her independence; her rejection of the tender gestures of her husband; of her need to have her own way.

The feelings of repugnance to sexual exchanges were interpreted as being the reawakened memories of her first frightening sexual experience. The findings at examination suggested that she needed someone to trust. The doctor said she had lost the trust which a child has and to be childlike again would be good.

At the next consultation the patient stated that sex though infrequent was no longer painful. She had begun to think about pregnancy and this surprised her. Then she suddenly became upset, saying 'You say I am not able to be weak and dependent but you do not know how I suffered in childhood. My father was angry; my mother scolding. I felt crushed and torn. Never do I wish to become a child again'.

It became apparent that the traumatic encounter at 15 years was not the first traumatic relationship but strongly reinforced an earlier one. In exploring her feelings with the therapist, the patient may have learnt that vulnerability does not always lead to pain and may have changed her feelings of distrust within her marriage.

Extracts from the film *Breaking the Ice*   Agnes Begg

Breaking the Ice — approaching sexual problems — was produced by the Edinburgh Human Sexuality Group who are involved in sexual counselling as well as teaching and training. The film is designed to assist in the training of doctors, nurses, social workers, clinical psychologists or, indeed, any health-care professional who is likely to meet a situation where patients with sexual difficulties seek advice. No attempt has been made in this film to provide solutions to psychosexual problems. A cameo is presented of a young couple who recognise they have a sexual problem but are unable to define clearly what that problem is. The ways in which the various professionals from whom they seek help deal with these patients, and how the patients relate to each other, are intended to provoke thoughts and questions about the fundamental need to communicate effectively in this important area of primary care.

Simply recognising this need is not of course, going to provide the solution to any psychosexual problem, since there are many barriers, attitudinal and social, to adequate communication, but it is hoped that the film will produce some understanding of what these barriers may be, and therefore be helpful in breaking them down.

Summaries

Genital pain in men   *D. C. MacDonald Burns*

Two cases were presented:

1. Man of 55, married with a grown-up daughter. Presented with pain in the penis, irritation between the legs, pain in the lower abdomen and at the top of his head. Strong feeling of guilt resulting from a suspected venereal infection 30 years previously in a casual relationship. He did then have a urethral discharge. Full investigations by a physician, neurologist and venereologist proved negative. Minimal improvement on anti-depressants. Further investigations by Dr Burns showed a prostatitis, diagnosed on prostatic massage. Treated with Co-trimixazole and referred back, because of the distance to his GP for follow-up.

2. Man of 45, overweight, complaining of perineal pain and altered unsatisfactory sensation at orgasm. History of vasectomy four years earlier. On examination found to have a circinate balanitis and evidence of a bacterial prostatitis on prostatic examination. Treatment of both conditions produced no improvement in his orgasmic problems.

Discussion
Physical and infective causes of pain in the perineal area should always be fully investigated and treated.

In the two cases presented the symptoms did not improve. It is probable that the guilt feelings in the first case should have been more deeply probed, including the underlying fears and fantasies. In the second case, could the vasectomy in association possibly with an extra-marital episode, have contributed to his orgasmic dissatisfaction?

Sexuality and body image   *Elsie Koadlow*

Sexual response may be dependent on a satisfactory body and genital image. This was illustrated by four cases.

Follow-up research in vaginismus after Masters & Johnson Therapy
H. Musaph

Forty-seven women treated for primary psychogenic vaginismus in the period 1975–78 were followed up in a pilot study. The mean time of treatment was 12–24 months. The patients were seen once a month.

A modified Masters & Johnson form of treatment was employed. Questionnaires were sent after completion of treatment to 47 couples. Twenty-three answered: 11 very satisfied; 7 satisfied; 2 not satisfied; 3 not at all satisfied.

Conclusions
(1) Failure to put the patient at ease during the vaginal examination. (2) Too much focus on reaching vaginal penetration and too little on non-genital sexuality. (3) Not enough emphasis on the importance of motivation, emotions and behaviour of the whole personality and the interaction with the partner.

The risks of oral and anal intercourse   *Jules S. Black*

Medical risks are infective or traumatic in origin:

Infection: (i) Fungal — Oral candida is the most significant — 40 per cent of the population carry the yeast as a normal mouth commensal. Recurrent vulvo-vaginitis may be caused by poor anal hygiene and ano-vaginal sex. (ii) Bacterial — neisserial, haemophilus especially in urinary infections. (iii) Viral — herpes. (iv) Miscellaneous microbial infections.

Trauma: Foreign bodies, finger nails with poor hygiene, after fellatio.

Director of Training's concluding remarks

Prudence Tunnadine

The papers you have heard here have been attempts to distil the findings of many hundreds of doctors over 25 years. Clearly it was not possible here to give much account of the method by which we arrived at them. I warned you in my introductory remarks that in the seminar discussions we could only hope to give you a flavour, and it is clear as we come to the end of the Conference, that some feel dissatisfaction that we have not spelled out our concepts of treatment.

This sense of dissatisfaction, this frustration that one has not received certainties, is common, not only to this Conference, but to any new doctor entering training in this subject. This is inevitable and to be respected, for the need for certainty, not only in our patients but in ourselves, in an area of our lives and work in which uncertainty is so threatening, is inescapable. Doctors, if they cannot remember a new drug, turn to the data compendium and look it up, without shame. But if patients seek our help with their sexual lives and we do not know the answer, we feel it reveals ignorance in our private selves. We should not despair; this is difficult for everybody. The essence of our training is not to aim for great knowledge of sexual matters — rather to conceptualise and improve our skills in dealing with our patients. Yet we should not be surprised that in our vulnerable sense of ignorance we turn to any magic routine that provides certainty, just as our patients demand of us any magic routine that will make their sexual performance easier. It is so much more difficult, more threatening, to have to look within ourselves be we patients or doctors. I cannot give you such certainty because the training of this Institute does not aim to turn out clones of Tom Main or even Pru Taunnadine, but rather to help each individual doctor to become conscious of his own clinical strength and weakness, style and prejudices and blind spots. Thus we begin gradually to sit back and think for ourselves. For example, one doctor may recognise that vasectomy gets his hackles up, another that he is in trouble when some rather 'tarty' patient makes him feel safer behind his desk than getting her on the couch to examine her. As we become aware of these facets in ourselves, we are enabled to see such an event in our clinical work, not as a threat, but as an interesting fact about the patient in front of us. The doctor who is not keen on vasectomy may notice that one patient gets his agreement despite his resistances, while the next patient makes him feel it is a good idea. Similarly one attractive women patient by the seductiveness of her behaviour threatens the other's ability to act as her doctor, and the next equally attractive patient gets him treating her protectively like a Dutch uncle — thus we begin to make dispassionate, factual observations about the effect patients have on us, and hence about the light that this throws upon their effect on other people and upon their sexual attitudes. These may be usefully interpreted to them so that they may recognise and review their less conscious attitudes towards their own sexuality and their partners.

Because this way of working is empirical, is not 'scientific' in terms of statistical analysis and measurable anatomy and physiology, is it invalid as a clinical science? I argue that in this most psychosomatic of all fields the one fact which is clinically true, the one certainty about human nature, is that everyone is different — that everyone is not only different from others, but different through life. Human sexuality and its relationships are dynamic. They change by the moment and by the moment they are changed. Both patient and doctor change between the beginning of a consultation and the end. If we can accept this — and training helps us to do so — then it can be actually a relief to recognise that the most we as doctors can do is to catch these moments as they fly. This may not be called 'scientific', but it may actually be true; and the generalisations that we make about human beings may be labelled 'scientific' but are by definition 'false'.

In traditional doctoring we have to know the answer: our way is 'normal' and right, and we teach our patients how to conform to the 'norm'. In my view that is inflicting personal views upon our patients rather than, as we try to do, helping them to find out what is right for themselves. We cannot, I believe, avoid the issue that there is an essential difference in motive between helping patients adapt to a 'norm' on the one hand, and helping them to find their own way on the other. Our clinical task is surely to make a diagnosis before we declare treatment. Penicillin is very useful for sore throats and plaster of paris for broken legs, but neither is much use for the other. It is our experience that when patients seek sexual help from a doctor they expect body care as well as emotional understanding. How then can we define this use of the doctor-patient relationship and the 'moment of truth'?

The doctor-patient relationship is what happens between us and our patients. Different patients have different effects upon us. The classic frigidity story of the sleeping beauty provides an illustration. She had loving parents who warned her against the dangers of penetrating objects. When she encountered the penetrating object she fell into a deep sleep and built a defensive forest around her and lay waiting until her parents were long dead. Prince Charming had to fight his way through the thicket and awaken her with his kiss. This is an assessment of the patients' atttitude that can be achieved in two ways. It can be achieved by taking a history; asking questions about their parents; about what they think about penetrating objects and why they defend themselves. Or we can consider it as something that is happening before our eyes in the consulting room. This girl is making me treat her protectively — what is it all about? She feels threatened by anticipation of vaginal examinaion — of a penetrating object — making difficulties for me of a unique kind. This patient expects *me* to do all the work; to fight my way through the thicket of her defences; seeing her sexuality as a passive business — her arousal is the responsibility of her Prince Charming, as though she has no part of it.

It is her own desires she fights, but the effect on us is the same as the effect on her partner who, like us, feels like a rapist in trying to overcome these defences. In traditional medicine we tend to regard a 'good' doctor-patient relation as one that is all sweetness and light, but that may be useless to a patient who needs to understand the fight within herself. With men patients likewise, with gentle giants, out of touch with their confident assertiveness, if we ask questions about their mother they will certainly reply that she was marvellous. But a patient may reveal how he deals with powerful women the moment he comes into the room. It is not easy for a man to come to a woman doctor, and I can assume he will regard me as a terrifying monster. If in this anxiety he copes with me by a Uriah Heep-like placation, 'Very good of you to give me your time doctor', I may usefully be able to interpret this. If such a man comes back to me later and feels able to say 'Well, that was a bloody waste of time', I know he has been helped. Thus the doctor-patient relation can be observed in seconds, in the course of our everyday hurried consultations. If we know who we are, we can make some judgements about how each patient uniquely deals with other people in their lives.

I would like to correct some misapprehensions about the 'moment of truth' in genital examination which have led to the idea that if other kinds of therapists do genital examinations, they can thus somehow show their patients how to do sex. This is nonsense — our findings about genital examination are of another order. Doctors find their own ways of making genital examination an unembarrassing business for their patients and for themselves. Our studies show that people, in this unguarded moment of the anticipation of revealing parts that are not called private for nothing, very often reveal their true anxiety. If we are not too busy 'putting them at ease', if we can just listen and be aware, they may reveal their innermost feelings at this moment. It is, for a woman, anticipation of penetration of a kind, not only of her body but of the part of her emotional self in relation to her sexuality which is also kept private. She may show us a reflection not only of her physical behaviour in intercourse, but also of a clear body-mind language. We find that when a woman says something verbally or non-verbally about her vagina, she is often also saying something about the inner sexual desiring woman in her. The woman who says 'Am I rather small, doctor?' may also be saying 'Am I too young'? or 'Is sexuality a dangerous damaging thing?' A woman who apologises for not having bathed may not only be concerned about infection, but may be speaking also about her sexuality as something meriting apology or requiring cleaning up for public view and sharing. It is the patients' reaction to the anticipation or threat of examination that interests us — we do not necessarily have to get them up on the couch. Our task is to think on their behalf about things of which they are not fully conscious themselves. Having thus used these moments as a diagnostic process we may usefully share our perceptions with them to enlighten them about their attitudes to their sexuality. Only if we have thus received from them some clear information about their misapprehensions about their bodily structures or their desires is it any use actually confronting them with the physical facts by examination, or by inviting them to examine themselves. One cannot 'reassure' unless one knows what is lacking assurance in the first place. Guesswork is not to be confused with diagnosis.

In the early days we believed that this 'moment of truth' in anticipation of genital examination only applied to women. Indeed we developed a theory as to why this was the case. The vagina, we thought, was a hidden mysterious 'do not touch' organ, in contrast to the penis whose purpose and pleasure potential were obvious and overt from the earliest years. But as more men sought help, we found that they too often revealed their true anxiety as they dropped their trousers in preparation for this potentially threatening procedure. Again, this is purely diagnostic observation. A young man who was being examined for sub-fertility, for example, had a large varicocoele, but what he said when he dropped his trousers was 'Does size matter, doctor?' Rather than succumb to the temptation to guess what he might mean, I said only 'How do you mean?', and out came a classic story of looking down on what he thought was a small penis from his great height in the changing room. He had no sexual difficulty until he had to perform by the chart, feeling like a stud animal, in order to conceive. By allowing him to elaborate on his fears of smallness, I was then able to reassure him factually. He regained his confidence and his wife conceived before he had his varicocoele operated on.

This technique is not magic; it is based upon the fact that only our individual patients know what is inside their heads. Training helps us to bear the uncertainty of not being all-knowing and to create an atmosphere in which they can tell us.

I am aware, since this Conference has been so intensive, that our training must seem very daunting. Hearing papers from highly specialised doctors, painstakingly gathered over 25 years of toil and puzzlement, it may be hard to recognise that even today, each of us goes into each new consultation with the same question mark as ever. Our training has enabled us to see open-mindedness as a rich therapeutic skill rather than as terrifying ignorance. The sort of case I value in a seminar of mine might begin: 'Something funny happened to me in the surgery last night. I was sitting there relieved that the last patient was coming in — I might actually get home for the World Cup after all — and just as she was leaving she turned and said "Oh, by the way, doctor, this irritation that I am feeling, could it be anything to do with my husband?" — and my heart sank'. This is what doctoring is like. This is what we study in seminars. We value the fact that we are feeling human beings, unable to deliver magic answers. We study our dealings with one patient after another; we begin to conceptualise our personal passions and prejudices and tastes and anxieties; and to value them as factual, clinical observations.

President's closing address

Tom Main

I had prepared a closing address but in the last hour two things happened which make me feel that a formal address is inappropriate: the first was Dr Tunnadine's remark about the importance of relating to people rather than to ideas; the second was the widespread curiosity at this Conference about the rules of the Institute. What were these rules? Why were they not fully disclosed? This curiosity set me thinking. Should I ignore it and deliver my prepared address simply because it was on the Conference programme? Or should I respond to the interest in rules? A few minutes ago I decided not to offer you my sample of a 'doctor-paper' relation but rather a sample of a doctor puzzled but yet attempting to respond to the communications of others, no matter how ill prepared he may feel.

The Institute has clear administrative rules, the usual ones any organisation is liable to have — about fees, qualifications, etc. — but so far as technical rules are concerned, the Institute is vague, I suppose irritatingly so. Those of you who suspect strong but hidden rules, may be right — and yet wrong. Right in that the Institute's work certainly studies technical rules; wrong in so far as technical rules are not mandates, but only tips, such as any coach gives to his trainees. One overriding tip can be expressed as follows — Thought is like wool: there is no substitute for it. There is an ethic inside the Institute that thinking is better than the swapping of beliefs. But there is also awareness of an ever-present danger about thinking — which is that conclusions once arrived at tend to be promoted from the status of ideas to the status of moralities. For example, the idea that it is more useful to interpret the discerned defences against impulses, than simply to point out the underlying impulses, can itself easily become a morality, a *rule*, e.g. 'It is always *right* to interpret defences, it is always *bad* to point only to hidden impulses'.

All rules limit the freedom of the individual but there are two kinds of rules. The first limits freedom in the interests of someone else — usually an authority: the second limits one's freedom in the interests of oneself. Broadly speaking these could be called super-ego rules and ego rules. A super-ego rule might be exemplified by a notice on a bathing beach which says 'Private Beach. No bathing allowed. Penalty for trespass £10'. The characteristics of this rule are: it is anonymous and benefits someone else — but who? You do not know; it makes no sense; you are allowed no choice in the interpretations of the rule; it does not benefit you at all; it is maintained by unvarying penalty with no allowances made for circumstances; last, it is liable to give rise to rebellious thoughts such as 'Well, if I came down here at night, no one would see me'. An example of the ego rule is the rule of the road —which in this country is 'drive on the left'. Those who decided this rule got no benefits from it — it was simply a decision made in the interests of everybody. The rule is self-maintaining and enlists the cooperation of everyone's common sense; it does not need policing, because everyone joins in; those who obey it, benefit from it; it is not maintained by fixed penalty, but rather by the reality of other drivers (if you doubt this try driving on the right); lastly it does not tempt rebellion. Those who drive on the right will not be punished by the courts, but by the consequences in reality.

The Institute has many technical rules, and endeavours to test and retest them — they must make common sense to the ego. They are discussable for reliability, and for their benefits to those in this field; that is to say they are simply working tips, not designed to make life easier but more true, more interesting. These technical tips are not aimed at obedience and conformity but at skill. If the technical tips — or rules — do not make common sense, the Institute members are quick to find this out and to regard a technical rule as inappropriate. The Institute does not offer ethics or moralities about what is the *right* thing to do in various situations and does not instruct on *correct* techniques, but it does seek thoughtful critical assessment of doctor-patient transactions.

Sadly, it is almost impossible for one human being to understand another except for a few moments at a time. Those who are gifted get nearest to it, but no one ever really fully understands another person. To pretend one knows what the trouble is, that one knows exactly what to do, is usually immodest, often dishonest, and always grandiose, but it is humanly understandable as a flight from the pains of ineptitude. For indeed it is painful to be inept — to tolerate one's own ignorance and uncertainty. Yet together the members of this Institute have found that tolerating one's own ineptitude and uncertainty in the hope that later phenomena may emerge and make sense is both more satisfying to the doctor and more useful to the patient than routine treatments which attempt to eliminate surface phenomena. To be ignorant but willing, to tolerate the fact that one does not understand, and to go on thinking without reference to authoritative theory or quick solutions is not easy.

There may be some who came to this Conference hoping that they might go away with some tips that would make their lives easier, i.e. practical short cuts. To those who came with such hopes I can only repeat that the gloomy news is that there is no Santa Claus. Indeed, no one is going to solve your clinical problems for you. At this point I am reminded of Freud's reply to a questioner who asked him why psychoanalysis took so long. Freud answered with the story of the man who set out with his wife in the car for an evening's entertainment. The wife said, as they got into the car 'Look, we are late. We have no time for short cuts'. In the face of our problems, life has hard rules of its own, and understanding is difficult, but if one sits down, listens and thinks, stands the uncertainty, and tries as long as possible, one can have some hope of understanding something of one's patient, and thus of offering to the patient the view of a thoughtful outsider. The remarkable effect on the patient of being only slightly understood is well known to all here. How many times in a lifetime does one get the feeling that one is fully understood?

None of these matters is the preserve of members of this Institute. All doctors have to face distress, sometimes intolerable, and to avoid being overwhelmed by it many of us adopt a defensive method of one sort or another; becoming conveniently blind or deaf if the topic is embarrassing, frightening or guilt-inducing; angry or apologetic if the patient's manner contains veiled threats; resigned and useless with castrative patients; or authoritarian in the face of the humble; and so on.

I have now moved from various defences that doctors adopt to avoid pain to the effects different patients have on doctors. The doctor should be alert not only about observing his characteristic responses to patients, but about the effect different patients have on him. He should not censor himself but value himself as a measuring instrument. If he feels angry that is a fact, a fact not for action or counter-anger, but a fact for cool observation and thought. Some patients make their doctors feel wonderful, others make their doctors feel useless, others make their doctors feel intellectually small. If the patient treats you as a magician and remarks upon your wisdom and ability, it is difficult to refuse this offer; but if you fall for it, it means that you have stopped thinking and have lost the chance of wondering what it is about this patient which requires him to praise his therapists, whether he has always had these tendences and how they operate in his daily life. This study of the doctor-patient relation can be informative about the responses the patient evokes in others in their environment.

246

And now for a rule — a technical tip. If the doctor feels something he should not act on it, but record that as a clinical fact which *may* throw some light on his patient. This rule is far from easy to follow; it is not a morality to be followed slavishly, but a practical tip for doctors to use in their own way.

This week members of the Institute have laid their work before the Conference and have shown the sort of thinking they have developed. You will agree with me that this thinking is by no means complete, but represents only the first fruits of a new approach. It comes from men and women who are prepared to account in seminars to their fellows about what they do; knowing it will be not only painful and sometimes humiliating but also useful in that they can have second thoughts about patients, a chance of thinking over their experience, and of learning from the experience of colleagues.

The training seminars themselves are therefore hard work and at times are depressing for the individual; they are suitable only for doctors who are modest enough to admit error and seek improvement of their skills. On the other hand it is comforting and exhilarating to be in the company of others in like case. At this point I would like to make it clear that the exposure and discussion of the personal styles of the doctors is limited to professional matters; the doctor's private neuroses are not discussed.

This is a body of people who are having a go and simply trying to get things right — we cannot preach at anyone, we have not made any great findings except that looking for the truth is difficult. We do not have a method of treatment, we simply have a way of looking and a way of thinking about the technique of being with patients — the listening method as compared with the telling method. I am saying these things emphatically because I really am very proud of the accomplishments of the people of this Institute, at the same time as I am highly critical of their defects. We just have to face the fact that none of us is good enough. I think that on that note I will just finish.

Appendix II

Index of papers from previous Conferences

The following papers were first printed for internal circulation in the *Proceedings of the Institute of Psychosexual Medicine's* annual conferences:

Bournemouth, 17-19 September, 1976
Anxiety and technique   *Alexandra Tobert*
Who is the patient?   *Ruth Skrine*
Frigid wives: a revised classification   *Margaret Blair and Jean Pasmore*
The doctor-patient relationship with men   *Prudence Tunnadine*

Durham, 9-11 September, 1977
Learning experience in a basic seminar   *Mary Rees and June Betts*
Learning in an advanced seminar   *Dorothy Morgan*
Working as a co-therapist   *Katharine Draper*

Cheltenham, 1-2 September, 1978
Vulnerability: a case study   *Joan R. Coombs*
Seminars and youth advisory work   *Gillian Hinshelwood*
The use of seminar training in general practice   *Peter Mitford*
Requests for abortion   *Ruth Coles*
Counselling in HM prisons   *Patricia Roberts*
The advantages of seminar training in a genetic counselling clinic *Elspeth M. Williamson*

Cheltenham, 6-7 October, 1979
Insights gained in seminars   *Doreen Anderson*
Insights gained in seminars   *Margaret Gill*
A cautionary tale   *Anne V. Smith*
Vasectomy counselling   *S. A. Corrin*
Psychosexual problems revealed during medical consultation requesting sterilisation   *James Bradshaw*

York, 13-14 September 1980
The use of Institute technique in marital therapy   *Jean Pasmore*
Defining the boundaries   *Margaret Blair*
Two case studies   *Alexandra Tobert*
The Institute and psychoanalysis   *Tom Main*

Cheltenham, 19-20 September 1981
Insights gained in seminars   *Elaine Cooper*
A case study concerning episiotomy   *Barbara Devereux*
A case study concerning an impotent diabetic   *Barbara Devereux*

248

The doctor-patient relationship in a man with recurrent pituitary adenoma   *Prudence Tunnadine*
Detecting psychosexual problems in the antenatal clinic   *James Bradshaw*
Psychosexual problems seen in the postnatal clinic   *Elizabeth Deman*
Care of patients with a known abnormal foetus   *Frank Johnson*

Three papers first appeared in the Institute's Newsletter:
Post-operative emotional problems with hysterectomy   *Prudence Tunnadine* (January 1977)
Psychosomatic pelvic pain   *Margaret Blair* (January 1978)
Reactions to rape   *Judy Gilley* (February 1979)

Appendix III

Institute of Psychosexual Medicine

The Institute of Psychosexual Medicine is a learned body for promotion of psychosexual medicine through seminar training and research.

It offers training to doctors to improve their skills with patients who seek help with sexual difficulties and related marital or psychosomatic problems, which may present openly or in the guise of other symptoms. Doctors who are suitable for this training thus work in general practice, family planning, community health, gynaecology, venerealogy, or psychiatry. The training aims to increase skill rather than knowledge, and the method of training is concerned with practice rather than theory. We do not try to change doctors into psychotherapists, but to develop their skills for managing psychosomatic problems.

Membership

Membership is limited to medical practitioners. There are the following categories:

a. Members

Doctors who have been passed by the Panel and been approved by Council.

b. Associate Members

Doctors who have been in training in an accredited seminar for at least two terms, but who have not yet been passed by the Panel. Associate Members can attend business meetings and receive the Newsletter, but have no vote.

c. Subscribers

Doctors working in the field of psychosexual medicine who apply to the Institute and are accepted by the Council although they have not had the formal Institute training. Subscribers can attend meetings and receive the Newsletter but have no vote.

Training

Basic Training Courses

Ten to 12 doctors meet fortnightly for two hours in terms of six sessions for two years. They treat their own patients from the start and report on their clinical consultations in continuing case discussions. These are supervised by a leader who is accredited by the Institute. The cases that are discussed are contraceptive problems; gynaecological or venerealogical problems with a psychosomatic element; requests for abortion or for sterilisation in men and women; menopausal and fertility problems; and difficulties with consummation, ejaculation, orgasm, and sexual enjoyment.

250

At the end of this course most doctors are able to diagnose these problems and to know which problems they can treat in their own clinical setting and in the time available, and when they should make an appropriate referral.

When a group of doctors want to meet together for this purpose the Institute will provide an accredited leader for them in most areas of the United Kingdom. Seminars may be recognised under Section 63 for General Practitioners.

Advanced Training

Doctors who seek to make this field a special interest, and who show aptitude, may be recommended by their basic seminar leader to proceed to further training as specialists in psychosexual medicine. After this they may offer themselves for examination by Panel and if successful are awarded the Institute's Certificate of Competence in Psychosexual Medicine. A doctor so qualified is competent to accept referrals from other practitioners and agencies.

Certificate of Competence

The criteria by which the Panel assess competence for qualification for specialist work.

i. An ability to understand genital examination as a psychosomatic event and to use these findings therapeutically.

ii. An ability to understand the contribution of both doctor and patient to the doctor-patient relationship.

iii. Sensitivity to unconscious elements in the patients' communications.

iv. Perception of the doctors' own individual strengths and weaknesses as clinicians.

v. Ability to select cases appropriate to this approach and to recognise unsuitable cases, such as those with deep seated pathology or personality disorders and those who cannot use interpretive therapy.

vi. Some knowledge of the psychodynamics of emotional development.

Meetings

Clinical meetings are held each year, and a residential weekend meeting outside London.

Newsletter

A newsletter is published twice a year, intended as the main instrument of communication between the scattered members.

Information

Applications from individual doctors, or from administrators who wish to inaugurate such training, general information about the Institute of Psychosexual Medicine and particulars of doctors qualified in psychosexual medicine may be obtained from the Institute of Psychosexual Medicine, 11 Chandos Street, London W1M 9DG. Tel: 01-580-1043

References

Starred titles are books recommended for further reading.

Balint, M. (1957): *The Doctor, his Patient and the Illness*. London: Pitman Medical Publishing.

Balint, M. & Balint, E. (1961): *Psychotherapeutic Technique in Medicine*. London: Tavistock Publications.

Bancroft, J. & Coles, L. (1976): Three years' experience in a sexual problem clinic. *Br. Med. J.* **1**, 1575–1577.

Begg, A. & Dickerson, M. (1980): A sexual problems clinic in a family planning centre. *Br. J. Fam. Plan.* **5**, 91–93.

Bischoff, R. (1975): Personal view. *Br. Med. J.* **4**, 755.

Blair, M. (1982): Charing Cross Fertility Control Symposium, 12–13 November, 1981. *Br. J. Clin. Pract.*, Symposium supplement 17.

Blair, M. & Pasmore, J. (1964): Frigid Wives. *Proceedings of the 6th International Congress of Psychotherapy*, 1964. Selected papers, pp. 1–7. Basel/New York: S. Karger.

Bramley, M. *et al.* (1981): Brief psychosomatic therapy for consumation of marriage. *Br. J. Obstet. Gynaec.* **88**, 819–824.

Burgess, A. & Holmstrom, L. (1974): Rape trauma syndrome. *Am. J. Psychiat.* **131**, 981–986.

Courtney, M. (1969): *Sexual Discord in Marriage*. London: Tavistock Publications.

*Freedman, R. (1983, in press): *Sexual Medicine*. London: Churchill Livingstone.

Friedman, L. T. (1962): *Virgin Wives*. London: Tavistock Publications.

Frommer, E. A. & O'Shea, G. (1973): Antenatal identification of women likely to have problems in managing their infants. *Br. J. Psychiat.* August, 123.

Frommer, E. A. & O'Shea, G. (1973): The importance of childhood experience in relation to problems of marriage and family building. *Br. J. Psychiat.*, August, 149–60.

Gilley, J. (1974): How to help the raped. *New Society*, 27 June.

Gilley, J. (1980): Help for women who have been raped. *Br. J. Fam. Plan.* **6**, 2.

Howard, G. (1978): Motivation for vasectomy. *Lancet* **1**, 546–548

Howard, G. (1979): The quality of marriage before and after vasectomy. *Br. J. Sex. Med.* **6**, 13, 14, 57.

Howard, G. (1980): Anxiety and neuroticism in couples requesting vasectomy. *Br. J. Fam. Plan.* **6**, 67–69.

Howard, G. (1982): Who asks for vasectomy reversal and why. *Br. Med. J.* **285**, 490–492.

Kaplan, H. S. (1974): *The New Sex Therapy*. London: Ballière Tindall.

*Lincoln, R. (1981): *Themes in Psychosexual Medicine*. Privately published by S. Phillips, Sutton, Surrey.

Main, T. F. (1966): Mutual projection in a marriage. *Comprehens. Psychiat.* **7**, 5.

Malan, D. H. (1979): *Individual Psychotherapy and the Science of Psychodynamics*. London: Butterworth.

Masters, W. H. & Johnson, V. E. (1966): *Human Sexual Response*. Boston: Little, Brown.

Masters, W. H. & Johsnon, V. E. (1970): *Human Sexual Inadequacy*. Boston, Little, Brown.

McCombie, S. (1975): Charcteristics of rape victims seen in crisis intervention. Published by The Rape Crisis Centre, PO Box 69, London WC1X 9NJ.

*Mears, E. (1978): Sexual problem clinics: an assessment of the work of 26 doctors trained by the Institute of Psychosexual Medicine. *Publ. Hlth., Lond.* **92**, 218–223.

Medea & Thompson, (1974): *Against Rape*. Noonday Press.

Rape Crisis Centre (1978, 1979): *Annual Reports*. Published by The Rape Crisis Centre, PO Box 69, London WC1X 9NJ.

Sutherland, S. & Scherl, D. (1970): Patterns of response amongst victims of rape. *Am. J. Orthopsychiat.* **40**, 503–511.

Tunnadine, L. D. P. (1970): *Contraception and Sexual Life*. London: Tavistock Publications.

*Tunnadine, L. P. D. (1983, in press): *The Making of Love. A Study of Individual Sexuality*. London: Jonathan Cape.

Index